A. J. Larner

# The 2x2 Matrix

Contingency, Confusion, and the Metrics
of Binary Classification

 Springer

A. J. Larner
Cognitive Function Clinic
Walton Centre for Neurology and Neurosurgery
Liverpool, UK

ISBN 978-3-030-74919-4          ISBN 978-3-030-74920-0   (eBook)
https://doi.org/10.1007/978-3-030-74920-0

This Springer imprint is published by the registered company Springer Nature Switzerland AG
The registered company address is: Gewerbestrasse 11, 6330 Cham, Switzerland

**To LF**
*Even in our deepest, most lasting friendships,
we never speak as openly as when we face a
blank page and address a reader we do not
know [Michel Houellebecq. Submission]*

# Preface

It is important to state at the outset what this book is not. It is not a textbook of medical statistics, as I have no training, far less any expertise, in that discipline. Rather it is a heuristic, based on experience of using and developing certain mathematical operations in the context of evaluating the outcomes of diagnostic and screening test accuracy studies. It therefore stands at the intersection of different disciplines, borrowing from them (a dialogic discourse?) in the hope that the resulting fusion or intermingling will result in useful outcomes. This reflects part of a wider commitment to interdisciplinary studies [6, 16].

Drawing as they do on concepts derived from decision theory, signal detection theory, and Bayesian methods, $2 \times 2$ contingency tables may find application in many areas, for example medical decision making, weather forecasting, information retrieval, machine learning and data mining. Of necessity, this volume is written from the perspective of the first of these areas, as the author is a practising clinician, but nevertheless it contains much material which will be of relevance to a wider audience.

Accordingly, this book is a distillate of what I have found to be helpful as a clinician working in the field of test accuracy studies, specifically related to the screening and diagnosis of dementia and cognitive impairment, undertaken in the context of a dedicated cognitive disorders clinic. The conceptual framework described here is supplemented with worked examples in each section of the book, over 60 in all, since, to quote Edwin Abbott, "An instance will do more than a volume of generalities to make my meaning clear" ([1], p. 56). Many of these examples are based on a large (N = 755) pragmatic prospective screening test accuracy study of one particular brief cognitive screening instrument, the Mini-Addenbrooke's Cognitive Examination (MACE) [3], the use of which in my clinical work has been extensively analysed and widely presented [7–9, 11–15]. (It has also been included in a systematic review of MACE [2].) Further analyses of MACE are presented here, along with material from some of the other studies which have been undertaken in the clinic [4]. My previous books documenting the specifics of such pragmatic test accuracy studies of cognitive screening instruments [5, 10] may be categorised as parerga, the current work being more general in scope and hence applicable to many branches of medical decision making as well as to disciplines beyond medicine wherein binary classification is required. Statistical programmes are not discussed.

James Clerk Maxwell (1831–1879) believed that there was "a department of the mind conducted independently of consciousness" where ideas could be "fermented and decocted so that when they run off they come clear" ([17], p. 94–5, 154), views with which I am largely in agreement (clarity of my own ideas, however, seldom being apparent). This prompts me to acknowledge two periods of annual leave, both spent at Center Parcs, Whinfell Forest, Cumbria, which lead to the embryonic over- all plan for this book (January 2019) and to the formulation of ideas about the epistemological matrix (November 2016).

Liverpool, UK                                                                                   A. J. Larner

# References

1. Abbott EA. Flatland. An edition with notes and commentary by William F Lindgren and Thomas F Banchoff. New York: Cambridge University Press/Mathematical Association of America; [1884] 2010.
2. Beishon LC, Batterham AP, Quinn TJ, et al. Addenbrooke's Cognitive Examination III (ACE-III) and mini-ACE for the detection of dementia and mild cognitive impairment. Cochrane Database Syst Rev. 2019;12:CD013282. [There are several numerical errors relating to my data in this publication, viz.: P7, Summary of findings: PPV for MCI vs. none incorrect for both 21 and 25 test threshold; P17, Figure 8: Incorrect N (= 754!), TP, FP, TN. Figure 9: Incorrect TP, FP, FN; P18, Figure 10: Incorrect N (= 756!), FP. Figure 11: Incorrect TP, FP, TN; P29, Characteristics of individual studies: "22 with MCI" should read "222 with MCI"; P52, Appendix 6, Summary of included studies: "DSM-V" should read "DSM-IV".]
3. Hsieh S, McGrory S, Leslie F, Dawson K, Ahmed S, Butler CR, et al. The Mini-Addenbrooke's Cognitive Examination: a new assessment tool for dementia. Dement Geriatr Cogn Disord. 2015;39:1–11.
4. Larner AJ. Dementia in clinical practice: a neurological perspective. Pragmatic studies in the Cognitive Function Clinic. 3rd edition. London: Springer; 2018.
5. Larner AJ. Diagnostic test accuracy studies in dementia: a pragmatic approach. 2nd edition. London: Springer; 2019.
6. Larner AJ. Neuroliterature. Patients, doctors, diseases. Literary perspectives on disorders of the nervous system. Gloucester: Choir Press; 2019.
7. Larner A. MACE: optimal cut-offs for dementia and MCI. J Neurol Neurosurg Psychiatry. 2019;90:A19.
8. Larner AJ. MACE for diagnosis of dementia and MCI: examining cut-offs and predictive values. Diagnostics (Basel). 2019;9:E51.
9. Larner AJ. Applying Kraemer's Q (positive sign rate): some implications for diagnostic test accuracy study results. Dement Geriatr Cogn Dis Extra. 2019;9:389–96.
10. Larner AJ. Manual of screeners for dementia. Pragmatic test accuracy studies. London: Springer; 2020.
11. Larner AJ. Screening for dementia: Q* index as a global measure of test accuracy revisited. medRxiv. 2020; https://doi.org/10.1101/2020.04.01.20050567.
12. Larner AJ. Defining "optimal" test cut-off using global test metrics: evidence from a cognitive screening instrument. Neurodegener Dis Manag. 2020;10:223–30.
13. Larner AJ. Mini-Addenbrooke's Cognitive Examination (MACE): a useful cognitive screening instrument in older people? Can Geriatr J. 2020;23:199–204.

14. Larner AJ. Assessing cognitive screening instruments with the critical success index. Prog Neurol Psychiatry. 2021;25(3):33–7.
15. Larner AJ. Cognitive testing in the COVID-19 era: can existing screeners be adapted for telephone use? Neurodegener Dis Manag. 2021;11:77–82.
16. Larner AJ. Neuroliterature 2. Biography, semiology, miscellany. Further literary perspectives on disorders of the nervous system. In preparation.
17. Mahon B. The man who changed everything. The life of James Clerk Maxwell. Chichester: Wiley; 2004.

# Acknowledgements

Thanks are due to Alison Zhu, a proper mathematician (1st in mathematics from Trinity College Cambridge) for advising on many of the equations in this book, although I hasten to add the any remaining errors are solely my own. Thanks also to Elizabeth Larner who drew Fig. 7.7.

# Contents

# Chapter 1
# Introduction

**Contents**

## 1.1 History and Nomenclature

Use of a fourfold or quadripartite 2 × 2 table to represent counts of different classes, a dichotomous classification, may date back to Aristotle [23]. Examples of the application of such tables to medical issues may be found in the work of Gavarret in the 1840s and Liebermeister in the 1870s [18, 23].

The term "contingency table" to describe a matrix format used to display a frequency distribution of variables is generally credited to Karl Pearson (1857–1936) in his lecture to the Draper's Society in 1904 [20]. Furthermore, in his book, *The grammar of science*, Pearson stated:

> … all we can do is to classify things into like within a certain degree of observation, and record whether what we note as following from them are like within another degree of observation. Whenever we do this … we really form a contingency table, … (cited from the 3rd edition of *The grammar of science* [18], pp.90–1).

Nevertheless, "contingency table" barely features in Porter's biography of Pearson ([21] p.266, 273).

The term "confusion matrix" or error matrix, or table of confusion, has also been applied to 2 × 2 tables, with the columns denoting instances of an actual class and the rows denoting instances of a predicted class. The term "confusion matrix" derives from the observation that this form of cross tabulation (or crosstab) makes it easy to see if the system is confusing two classes. The confusion matrix may be

© Springer Nature Switzerland AG 2021
A. J. Larner, *The 2x2 Matrix*, https://doi.org/10.1007/978-3-030-74920-0_1

described as a special kind (2 × 2) of contingency table, since higher order contingency tables may be constructed, cross tabulating instances into more classes, represented by more columns and/or rows (see Sect. 7.3.1). Another term sometimes used to describe the 2 × 2 table is a "truth table", by analogy with those tables developed by Ludwig Wittgenstein (1889–1951) for use in logic (see Sects. 1.3.1 and 7.3.4).

The 2 × 2 contingency table or confusion matrix hence reifies a binary system of classification. This should not, however, be confused with the binary or dyadic notation, using the base 2, the development of which is often associated (perhaps unjustifiably) with Gottfried Leibniz (1646–1716) [3].

The 2 × 2 contingency table is applicable to decision making in many disciplines. The details of this table are now described.

## 1.2   The Fourfold (2 × 2) Contingency Table

The simple 2 × 2 contingency table or confusion matrix cross-tabulates all instances (N) into classes, according to some form of reference standard or "true status" (e.g. diagnosis, or meteorological observations) in the vertical columns, against the outcome of a test or classifier of interest (e.g. a diagnostic or screening test, or meteorological forecasts) in the horizontal rows. In other words, there is a mapping of all instances to predicted classes, giving an indication of the performance of the classifier. The columns may be characterised as explanatory variables, the rows as response variables.

This quadripartite classification thus categorises all individuals, observations, or events as:

- true positive (TP), or "hits"
- false positive (FP), or "false alarms" or "false hits"
- false negative (FN), or "misses"
- true negative (TN), or "non events" or "correct rejections"

This cross-classification is shown in a 2 × 2 contingency table in Fig. 1.1. Henceforward the terms TP, FP, FN, TN will be referred to as "literal notation", and metrics derived from the 2 × 2 contingency table and denoted by equations using this notation as "literal equations". Some readers may find such literal terminology easier to use and comprehend than algebraic notation.

The 2 × 2 table is often set out using algebraic terms, where:

- TP = a
- FP = b
- FN = c
- TN = d

This is shown in Fig. 1.2. Henceforward the terms a, b, c, d will be referred to as "algebraic notation", and equations using this notation as "algebraic equations".

**Fig. 1.1**  2 × 2 contingency table using literal notation

| | | Condition present | Condition absent |
|---|---|---|---|
| | | **True Status** | |
| **Test Outcome** | **Positive** | True positive [TP] | False positive [FP] |
| | **Negative** | False negative [FN] | True negative [TN] |

**Fig. 1.2**  2 × 2 contingency table using algebraic notation

| | | Condition present | Condition absent |
|---|---|---|---|
| | | **True Status** | |
| **Test Outcome** | **Positive** | True positive (a) | False positive (b) |
| | **Negative** | False negative (c) | True negative (d) |

Some readers may find this algebraic terminology easier to use and comprehend than literal notation.

N is used throughout this book to denote the total number of instances observed or counted (e.g. patients or observations), in other words a population, such that:

$$N = TP + FP + FN + TN$$
$$= a + b + c + d$$

It should be noted, however, that some authors have used N to denote total negatives or negative instances (FN + TN, or c + d), for which the term $q'$ is used here (see Sect. 1.3.1).

## 1.3   Marginal Totals and Marginal Probabilities

### *1.3.1   Marginal Totals*

It is immediately obvious that the four cells of the 2 × 2 table will generate six marginal values or totals by simple addition in the vertical, horizontal, and diagonal directions (Fig. 1.3). These totals will be denoted here using lower case letters.

| | | True Status | | |
|---|---|---|---|---|
| | | **Condition present (= case)** | **Condition absent (= non case)** | r′ |
| **Test Outcome** | **Positive** | True positive [TP] (a) | False positive [FP] (b) | q |
| | **Negative** | False negative [FN] (c) | True negative [TN] (d) | q′ |
| | | p | p′ | r |

**Marginal totals:**

| | | | | |
|---|---|---|---|---|
| p | = | TP + FN | = | a + c |
| p′ | = | FP + TN | = | b + d |
| p + p′ | = | N | = | a + b + c + d |
| | | | | |
| q | = | TP + FP | = | a + b |
| q′ | = | FN + TN | = | c + d |
| q + q′ | = | N | = | a + b + c + d |
| | | | | |
| r | = | TP + TN | = | a + d |
| r′ | = | FP + FN | = | b + c |
| r + r′ | = | N | = | a + b + c + d |

**Marginal probabilities:**

| | | | | |
|---|---|---|---|---|
| P | = | (TP + FN)/N | = | p/N |
| (1 − P) = P′ | = | (FP + TN)/N | = | p′/N |
| | | | | |
| Q | = | (TP + FP)/N | = | q/N |
| (1 − Q) = Q′ | = | (FN + TN)/N | = | q′/N |
| | | | | |
| R | = | (TP + TN)/N | = | r/N |
| (1 − R) = R′ | = | (FP + FN)/N | = | r′/N |

**Fig. 1.3**  $2 \times 2$ contingency table with marginal totals and marginal probabilities

Reading vertically, down the columns:

$$p \quad = \quad TP + FN \quad = \quad a + c$$
$$p' \quad = \quad FP + TN \quad = \quad b + d$$

$$p + p' \quad = \quad N$$

**Fig. 1.4** 2 × 2 truth table
for "p" and "not p" (or
"–p")

| | | Criterion diagnosis | |
|---|---|---|---|
| | | **D+** | **D-** |
| Classifier diagnosis | **D+** | True | False |
| | **D-** | False | True |
| | | p | p' |

In other words, p = positive instances and p′ = negative instances. This may also be illustrated in a simple truth table akin to that used in logic when using "p" and "–p" or "not p" for propositions (Fig. 1.4).

A dataset is said to be balanced when p = p′. A difference in these columnar marginal totals (i.e. in the numbers of positive, p, and negative, p′, instances) is termed class imbalance. This may impact on the utility of some measures derived from the 2 × 2 contingency table.

Reading horizontally, across the rows:

$$q \quad = \quad TP + FP \quad = \quad a + b$$
$$q' \quad = \quad FN + TN \quad = \quad c + d$$

$$q + q' \quad = \quad N$$

In other words, q = positive classifications and q′ = negative classifications. It is also possible to read the table diagonally:

$$r \quad = \quad TP + TN \quad = \quad a + d$$
$$r' \quad = \quad FP + FN \quad = \quad b + c$$

$$r + r' \quad = \quad N$$

In other words, r = true instances and r′ = false instances. (It should be noted that the use of "r" here has a different meaning from that used by other authors with respect to ratios of relevant costs, and in kappa values.)

Henceforward the terms p, p′, q, q′, r, r′ will be referred to as marginal totals and will be substituted in some algebraic equations.

### 1.3.2   Marginal Probabilities; P, Q

The six absolute marginal totals may be converted to six probabilities, or rates, by dividing each by N. These probabilities or rates will be denoted using upper case letters.

Reading vertically in Fig. 1.3:

$$P \quad = \quad (TP+FN)/N \quad = \quad (a+c)/N \quad = \quad p/N$$
$$P' = (1-P) \quad = \quad (FP+TN)/N \quad = \quad (b+d)/N \quad = \quad p'/N$$

As probabilities, these values necessarily sum to unity:

$$P+P' \quad = \quad 1$$

P is the prevalence, or prevalence rate, or base rate. When P = 0.5 there is a balanced class distribution (i.e. no class imbalance) because by definition P' = 0.5.

P is used throughout this book to denote prevalence. It should be noted, however, that some authors use P to denote total positives or positive instances (TP + FP, or a + b), for which the term q is used here (Sect. 1.3.1).

Prevalence may also be expressed in probability notation, as the probability that disease is either present, the pre-test probability, $p(D+)$, or absent, $p(D-)$.

**Worked Example: Prevalence Rates (P, P')**
The Mini-Addenbrooke's Cognitive Examination (MACE) [8], a brief cognitive screening instrument, was subjected to a screening test accuracy study in a large patient cohort, N = 755 [11]. A reference (criterion) diagnosis of dementia, based on the application of widely accepted diagnostic criteria for dementia, was made in 114 patients. At the MACE cut-off of ≤20/30, the test outcomes were as follows: TP = 104, FN =10, FP = 188, and TN = 453.

Hence the prevalence (P) or pre-test probability of dementia patients in this cohort was:

$$P \quad = \quad (TP+FN)/N$$
$$= \quad (104+10)/755$$
$$= \quad 0.151$$
$$= \quad p(D+)$$

The prevalence (P′) of patients without dementia, or pre-test probability against dementia, in the cohort was:

$$
\begin{aligned}
P' &= (FP+TN)/N \\
&= (188+453)/755 \\
&= 0.849 \\
&= 1-P \\
&= p(D-)
\end{aligned}
$$

Prevalence may be a useful estimate of pre-test probability (see also Sect. 4.7) from which pre-test odds may be calculated (Sect. 1.3.3). However, sample prevalence may differ from population prevalence, and hence this base rate may be no more than an anchor from which to make adjustments. Many of the measures derived from the $2 \times 2$ contingency table may be dependent on prevalence. This variation may be examined empirically, for example by using patient cohorts with different base rates of disease prevalence (e.g. [14, 15, 24], and [16], p.160,165) or by calculation at fixed values of prevalence (Sect. 2.3.2) (e.g. [11, 16]).

Reading horizontally in Fig. 1.3:

$$
Q = (TP+FP)/N = (a+b)/N = q/N
$$

Hence Q may be described as the positive sign rate [9] or the probability of a positive test in the study population.

$$
Q' = (1-Q) = (FN+TN)/N = (c+d)/N = q'/N
$$

Hence Q′ may be described as the negative sign rate [12] or the probability of a negative test in the study population.

$$
Q+Q' = 1
$$

Q may also be expressed in probability notation, as the probability that the test is either positive, $p(T+)$, or negative, $p(T-)$.

**Worked Example: Positive and Negative Sign Rates (Q, Q')**
In the screening test accuracy study of (MACE) [11], from the patient cohort
(N = 755) at the MACE cut-off of ≤20/30, the test outcomes were as follows:
TP = 104, FN =10, FP = 188, and TN = 453.
Hence the positive sign rate (Q) at MACE cut-off ≤20/30 was:

$$
\begin{aligned}
Q &= (TP + FP)/N \\
&= (104 + 188)/755 \\
&= 0.387 \\
&= p(T+)
\end{aligned}
$$

The negative sign rate (Q') at this cut-off was:

$$
\begin{aligned}
Q' &= (FN + TN)/N \\
&= (10 + 453)/755 \\
&= 0.613 \\
&= 1 - Q \\
&= p(T-)
\end{aligned}
$$

Many of the measures derived from the 2 × 2 contingency table may be dependent on level of the test, Q, evident as variation with test cut-off. Looking at Q is one
of the recommended steps in designing, conducting, reporting, and interpreting
receiver operating characteristic (ROC) analyses to support clinical decision making ([25], p.205) (see Sect. 6.2).

Reading the main diagonal (upper left to lower right) in Fig. 1.3:

$$
R = (TP + TN)/N = (a + d)/N = r/N
$$

Reading the off diagonal (lower left to upper right) in Fig. 1.3:

$$
R' = (1 - R) = (FP + FN)/N = (b + c)/N = r'/N
$$

$$
R + R' = 1
$$

R is sometimes known as "proportion correct" or "true rate" or accuracy (Sect.
3.2.4), and R' as "proportion incorrect" or "false rate" or misclassifications or inaccuracy or error rate (Sect. 3.2.4).

**Worked Example: Proportions Correct and Incorrect (R, R′)**
In the screening test accuracy study of (MACE) [11], from the patient cohort
(N = 755), at the MACE cut-off of ≤20/30, the test outcomes were as follows:
TP = 104, FN =10, FP = 188, and TN = 453.
  Hence the proportion correct (R) at MACE cut-off ≤20/30 was:

$$
\begin{aligned}
R &= (TP+TN)/N \\
&= (104+453)/755 \\
&= 0.737
\end{aligned}
$$

The proportion incorrect (R′) at this cut-off was:

$$
\begin{aligned}
R' &= (FP+FN)/N \\
&= (188+10)/755 \\
&= 0.263 \\
&= 1-R
\end{aligned}
$$

### 1.3.3   Pre-test Odds

Pre-test odds are given by the ratio of prevalence (or pre-test probability; Sect.
1.3.2) of instances with and without the item of interest (e.g. diagnosis, observation):

$$
\begin{aligned}
\text{Pre-test odds} &= P/(1-P) \\
&= P/P'
\end{aligned}
$$

In probability notation:

$$
\text{Pre-test odds} = p(D+)/p(D-)
$$

These are the odds favouring an event. Odds against the event are given by:

$$
\begin{aligned}
\text{Pre-test odds against} &= (1-P)/P \\
&= P'/P
\end{aligned}
$$

In probability notation:

$$
\text{Pre-test odds against} = p(D-)/p(D+)
$$

The pre-test odds can be simply converted to pre-test probability:

**Worked Example: Pre-test Odds for and against**
In the screening test accuracy study of (MACE) [11], in the total patient cohort (N = 755) the prevalence of dementia (P) was 0.151 and the prevalence of the absence of dementia (1 − P) was therefore 0.849.

Hence the pre-test odds of dementia were:

$$
\begin{aligned}
\text{Pre-test odds} \ &= \ P/(1-P) \\
&= \ 0.151/0.849 \\
&= \ 0.178
\end{aligned}
$$

The pre-test odds against dementia were:

$$
\begin{aligned}
\text{Pre-test odds against} \ &= \ (1-P)/P \\
&= \ 0.849/0.151 \\
&= \ 5.62
\end{aligned}
$$

$$
\text{Pre-test probability} \ = \ \text{Pre-test odds}/(1+\text{Pre-test odds})
$$

$$
\text{Pre-test probability} \ = \ 1/(1+\text{Pre-test odds against})
$$

Comparison of pre-test odds and post-test odds may be used in the Bayesian evaluation of tests (see Sect. 2.3.5). These odds also have a role in combining test results (Sect. 7.3.4).

## 1.4   Type I ($\alpha$) and Type II ($\beta$) Errors

A variant of the simple $2 \times 2$ contingency table may be constructed which cross-classifies all instances (N) according to the outcome of the null hypothesis (Fig. 1.5), since this leads to a binary outcome (reject or do not reject). Here, the "true status" (vertical columns) refers to whether the null hypothesis is true or false, whilst the "test outcome" (horizontal rows) refers to whether or not the null hypothesis is rejected.

Type I (or $\alpha$) error rate is the probability of rejecting the null hypothesis when in reality the null hypothesis is true; in other words detecting an effect that does not exist (false positive), an error of commission.

Type II (or $\beta$) error rate, sometimes denoted power, is the probability of not rejecting the null hypothesis when it is in reality false (false negative); in other words failing to detect an effect that does exist, an error of omission.

| | | True Status | |
|---|---|---|---|
| | | **Null hypothesis false** | **Null hypothesis true** |
| **Test Outcome** | **Reject null** | Correct: $1 - \beta$, power | Type I error: $\alpha$, false positive |
| | **Fail to reject null** | Type II error: $\beta$, false negative | Correct: $1 - \alpha$ |

**Fig. 1.5**   $2 \times 2$ table using error notation

These terms may be rearranged, such that $1 - \beta$ is the probability of rejecting the null hypothesis when it is false, or $\beta = (1 - \text{power})$.

- Null hypothesis false, rejected (i.e. correct) $= 1 - \beta$ ("power")
- Null hypothesis true, rejected $= \alpha$ (false positive, type I error)
- Null hypothesis false, fail to reject $= \beta$ (false negative, type II error)
- Null hypothesis true, fail to reject (i.e. correct) $= 1 - \alpha$

It should be noted that the four cells here are not equivalent to the four cells in the simple $2 \times 2$ table (Figs. 1.1 and 1.2).

Testing the null hypothesis by calculating $p$ values is fraught with the possibility of drawing incorrect conclusions. The conventional tendency to "dichotomise" $p$ values as significant or non-significant at the 0.05 level risks both type I ($p < 0.05$ may be a false positive) and type II ($p > 0.05$ may be a false negative) errors [2].

Henceforward the terms $1 - \beta$, $\alpha$, $\beta$, $1 - \alpha$ will be referred to as "error notation", and equations using this notation as "error equations".

## 1.5    Calibration: Decision Thresholds or Cut-Offs

When constructing a $2 \times 2$ contingency table, test outcome may be obvious (e.g. a clinical sign is either present or absent, a forecast was either made or not made). Sometimes, however, the classification is not binary or categorical, for example when using tests with a quantitative range of scores or continuous values. Measurement scales may be classified in various ways, with one system distinguishing between those scales with variables in ordered categories the distances between which either have the same meaning (linear; interval data) or have different or unknown meaning (non-linear; ordinal data) [22]. Many scales used in clinical practice are ordinal in nature [16].

For the purposes of constructing a 2 × 2 contingency table using quantitative scales, there is a need to dichotomise results according to a chosen threshold, also variously known as a cut-off, cut-point, decision threshold, dichotomisation point, or positivity criterion. For some tests, cut-off point(s) may be specified, for example in the test manual or in the index publication. However, these may not be readily transferable to other study populations. Defining the optimal cut-off(s) may be achieved by various methods ([13], p.36–41, [17]) (see Sect. 6.2), although it has been argued that cut-offs should not be determined post hoc as this risks introducing bias into study results [6]. This calibration process, the setting of the decision threshold(s) or cut-off(s), so that tests which produce continuous scale data may be used as if they were binary classifiers, will affect many of the outcome measures of a 2 × 2 contingency table. The setting of a cut-off will determine the level of the test, Q (Sect. 1.3.2).

The shortcomings of such dichotomisation are recognised: greater statistical power is afforded by the continuous approach [1, 5]. However, in clinical practice such dichotomisation is often pragmatic. Clinicians (and indeed patients) may generally be said to prefer binary classifiers (e.g. screen positive vs screen negative; target diagnosis present vs absent) since their categorical nature gives an impression of certainty and clarifies whether or not a medical intervention is applied.

## 1.6   Uncertain or Inconclusive Test Results

There are potential problems with the use of dichotomous thresholds. Things which once appeared or were conceptualised as binary or dimorphic may prove to be part of a spectrum or continuum (e.g. consciousness, sexuality). Disease entities once codified as binary may subsequently be recognised as spectrum disorders (e.g. Alzheimer's disease, compare diagnostic criteria of 1984 [19] and 2014 [7]). Providing a single cut-off score may therefore risk misclassifications. Indeed some authors advocate the abandonment of binary disease categories in favour of a probability dysfunction model based on risk of harm according to risk banding [4].

Three-way classification, or trichotomisation, has been suggested as a method to allow better classification accuracy but at the cost of not classifying a proportion of cases. Specifically, uncertain test scores, the most error-prone, are excluded or deselected from classification. This may be a substantial proportion of the test cohort, particularly if the test has limited strength, with unclassified individuals requiring further assessment for correct classification, achieved either by watchful waiting/ active surveillance or by the application of further (more sophisticated, more expensive, more risky) tests [10].

Higher order contingency tables (2 × 3, 2 × 4, 3 × 3) may also be a method to handle problems of this kind (Sect. 7.3.1).

## 1.7 Measures Derived from a 2 × 2 Contingency Table; Confidence Intervals

Aside from the marginal totals and probabilities (Sect. 1.3), a large number of other measures may be derived from a 2 × 2 contingency table. Many of these measures will be described in the subsequent chapters of this book, including but not limited to sensitivity and specificity, predictive values, and likelihood ratios. None is perfect, all have potential shortcomings, as well as utilities, in describing the outcomes of a contingency table. Indeed, it might be intuited that the very multiplicity of these measures suggests their inadequacy: all summary statistics reduce the information to a single characteristic of the data. (Perhaps a vector in the unit 4-dimensional space of a hypercube or tesseract might be a unique outcome descriptor for each 2 × 2 table, and be a potential comparator measure, but whether this would prove readily applicable, particularly in clinical practice, is highly questionable.)

To account for sampling variability, calculation of confidence intervals (or compatibility intervals) for each point estimate is recommended as a measure of precision. This quantification of statistical uncertainty is typically expressed using the 95% confidence interval (95% CI), in other words one can be 95% certain that the true value lies between these limits. Narrow confidence intervals (greater precision) result from large sample sizes, whereas small sample sizes may be associated with broad confidence intervals (lesser precision, hence more often give extreme results). Failure to quote confidence intervals may influence the generalizability of diagnostic studies ([13], p.53–4).

## References

1. Altman DG, Royston P. The cost of dichotomising continuous variables. Br Med J. 2006;332:1080.
2. Amrhein V, Greenland S, McShane B. Scientists rise up against statistical significance. Nature. 2019;567:305–7.
3. Ares J, Lara J, Lizcano D, Martinez MA. Who discovered the binary system and arithmetic? Did Leibniz plagiarize Caramuel? Sci Eng Ethics. 2018;24:173–88.
4. Baum ML. The neuroethics of biomarkers. What the development of bioprediction means for moral responsibility, justice, and the nature of mental disorder. Oxford, Oxford University Press; 2016.
5. Cohen J. The cost of dichotomization. Appl Psychol Meas. 1983;7:249–53.
6. Davis DH, Creavin ST, Noel-Storr A, et al. Neuropsychological tests for the diagnosis of Alzheimer's disease dementia and other dementias: a generic protocol for cross-sectional and delayed-verification studies. Cochrane Database Syst Rev. 2013;3:CD010460.
7. Dubois B, Feldman HH, Jacova C, et al. Advancing research diagnostic criteria for Alzheimer's disease: the IWG-2 criteria. Lancet Neurol. 2014;13:614–29. [Erratum Lancet Neurol. 2014;13:757]
8. Hsieh S, McGrory S, Leslie F, Dawson K, Ahmed S, Butler CR, et al. The Mini-Addenbrooke's Cognitive Examination: a new assessment tool for dementia. Dement Geriatr Cogn Disord. 2015;39:1–11.

9. Kraemer HC. Evaluating medical tests. Objective and quantitative guidelines. Newbery Park: Sage; 1992.

10. Landsheer JA. The clinical relevance of methods for handling inconclusive medical test results: quantification of uncertainty in medical decision-making and screening. Diagnostics (Basel). 2018;8:32.

11. Larner AJ. MACE for diagnosis of dementia and MCI: examining cut-offs and predictive values. Diagnostics (Basel). 2019;9:E51.

12. Larner AJ. Applying Kraemer's Q (positive sign rate): some implications for diagnostic test accuracy study results. Dement Geriatr Cogn Dis Extra. 2019;9:389–96.

13. Larner AJ. Diagnostic test accuracy studies in dementia. A pragmatic approach. 2nd ed. London: Springer; 2019.

14. Larner AJ. The "attended alone" and "attended with" signs in the assessment of cognitive impairment: a revalidation. Postgrad Med. 2020;132:595–600.

15. Larner AJ. Mini-Addenbrooke's Cognitive Examination (MACE): a useful cognitive screening instrument in older people? Can Geriatr J. 2020;23:199–204.

16. Larner AJ. Manual of screeners for dementia. Pragmatic test accuracy studies. London: Springer; 2020.

17. Larner AJ. Defining "optimal" test cut-off using global test metrics: evidence from a cognitive screening instrument. Neurodegener Dis Manag. 2020;10:223–30.

18. Matthews JR. Quantification and the quest for medical certainty. Princeton University Press: Princeton; 1995.

19. McKhann G, Drachman D, Folstein M, Katzman R, Price D, Stadlan EM. Clinical diagnosis of Alzheimer's disease. Report of the NINCDS-ADRDA work group under the auspices of the Department of Health and Human Service Task forces on Alzheimer's disease. Neurology. 1984;34:939–44.

20. Pearson K. Draper's company research memoirs. Biometric series I. Mathematical contributions to the theory of evolution XIII. On the theory of contingency and its relation to association and normal correlation. London: Dulau & Co.; 1904.

21. Porter TM. Karl Pearson: the scientific life in a statistical age. Princeton/Oxford: Princeton University Press; 2004.

22. Stevens SS. On the theory of scales of measurement. Science. 1946;103:677–80.

23. Stigler S. The missing early history of contingency tables. Ann Fac Sci Toulouse. 2002;11:563–73.

24. Wojtowicz A, Larner AJ. Diagnostic test accuracy of cognitive screeners in older people. Prog Neurol Psychiatry. 2017;21(1):17–21.

25. Youngstrom EA. A primer on receiver operating characteristic analysis and diagnostic efficiency statistics for pediatric psychology: we are ready to ROC. J Pediatr Psychol. 2014;39:204–21.

# Chapter 2
# Paired Measures

## Contents

## 2.1   Introduction

Several paired measures may be derived from the basic $2 \times 2$ contingency table. The classification of these measures as error-based, information-based, and association-based, following Bossuyt [2], is used in this chapter. Other classifications might have been used, such as test-oriented measures (e.g. sensitivity and specificity, false positive and false negative rates, likelihood ratios) versus patient-oriented measures (predictive values, predictive ratios).

## 2.2  Error-Based Measures

### 2.2.1  Sensitivity (Sens) and Specificity (Spec), or True Positive and True Negative Rates (TPR, TNR)

Yerushalmy [36] and Neyman [30] are usually credited as the first authors to discuss the statistical aspects of screening and diagnostic tests, and Yerushalmy introduced the terms sensitivity (Sens) and specificity (Spec) to denote respectively the inherent ability of a test to detect correctly a condition when it is present and to rule it out correctly when it is absent. Sens and Spec are conditional probabilities with range from 0 to 1, with higher values better. They are "uncalibrated measures of test quality ... with a variable zero-point and scale" ([14], p.65). There is a trade-off between Sens and Spec, since as the value of one rises the other falls.

Sensitivity (Sens) is sometimes known as true positive rate or ratio (TPR), hit rate, recall, or success ratio. In medical practice it is the probability of a positive test given the presence of disease, or the proportion of test positivity in the presence of a target condition, hence more generally a positive classification by the test in the presence of a given class.

In literal notation (Fig. 2.1):

$$\text{Sens} \quad = \quad \text{TP} / (\text{TP} + \text{FN})$$

or, with marginal total notation:

$$\text{Sens} \quad = \quad \text{TP} / \text{p}$$

In algebraic notation:

$$\begin{aligned} \text{Sens} \quad &= \quad a / (a + c) \\ &= \quad a / p \end{aligned}$$

In error notation (see Fig. 1.5):

$$\text{Sens} \quad = \quad (1 - \beta)$$

Sens may also be expressed in probability notation. If a test may be either positive, T+, or negative, T−, when used to distinguish between the presence, D+, or absence, D−, of a target disease, then:

$$\text{Sens} \quad = \quad p(\text{T+} \mid \text{D+})$$

Specificity (Spec) is sometimes known as true negative rate or ratio (TNR). In medical practice it is the probability of a negative test given the absence of disease, or the proportion of test negativity among the healthy, hence more generally a negative classification by the test in the absence of a given class. Hence both Sens and Spec are test-oriented measures.

| | | True Status | | |
|---|---|---|---|---|
| | | **Condition present** (= case) | **Condition absent** (= non case) | r′ |
| **Test Outcome** | **Positive** | True positive [TP] (a) | False positive [FP] (b) | q |
| | **Negative** | False negative [FN] (c) | True negative [TN] (d) | q′ |
| | | p | p′ | r |

**Paired measures (algebraic notation only):**

| | | | | |
|---|---|---|---|---|
| Sens (TPR) | = | a/(a + c) | | |
| Spec (TNR) | = | d/(b + d) | | |
| FPR | = | (1 − Spec) | = | b/(b + d) |
| FNR | = | (1 − Sens) | = | c/(a + c) |
| PPV | = | a/(a + b) | | |
| NPV | = | d/(c + d) | | |
| FDR | = | (1 − PPV) | = | b/(a + b) |
| FRR | = | (1 − NPV) | = | c/(c + d) |
| LR+ | = | TPR/(1 − TNR) | = | [a/(a + c)]/[b/(b + d)] |
| LR− | = | (1 − TPR)/TNR | = | [c/(a + c)]/[d/(b + d)] |
| DOR | = | LR+/LR− | = | ad/bc |
| EOR | = | ab/cd | | |
| CUI+ | = | Sens x PPV | = | a/(a + c) x a/(a + b) |
| CUI− | = | Spec x NPV | = | d/(b + d) x d/(c + d) |

**Fig. 2.1** 2 × 2 contingency table with literal and algebraic notation, marginal totals, and derived paired measures

**Worked Example: Sens, Spec**
The Mini-Addenbrooke's Cognitive Examination (MACE) [11] was subjected to a screening test accuracy study in a large patient cohort, N = 755 [15]. At the MACE cut-off of ≤20/30, the test outcomes for the diagnosis of dementia were as shown in the 2 × 2 contingency table (Fig. 2.2): TP = 104, FN = 10, FP = 188, and TN = 453.

|                     | Diagnosis |  |
|---------------------|-------------------|-------------------|
|                     | **Dementia present** | **Dementia absent** |
| MACE  ≤20/30 Outcome | True positive [TP] = **104** | False positive [FP] = **188** |
|        >20/30        | False negative [FN] = **10** | True negative [TN] = **453** |

**Fig. 2.2**  2 × 2 contingency table for Mini-Addenbrooke's Cognitive Examination (MACE) outcomes (N = 755) for the diagnosis of dementia at MACE cut-off of ≤20/30. (Data from [15])

Hence the values for Sens and Spec at this cut-off are:

$$\begin{aligned} \text{Sens} &= \text{TP} / (\text{TP} + \text{FN}) \\ &= 104 / (104 + 10) \\ &= 0.912 \end{aligned}$$

$$\begin{aligned} \text{Spec} &= \text{TN} / (\text{FP} + \text{TN}) \\ &= 453 / (188 + 453) \\ &= 0.707 \end{aligned}$$

In literal notation:

$$\begin{aligned} \text{Spec} &= \text{TN} / (\text{FP} + \text{TN}) \\ &= \text{TN} / p' \end{aligned}$$

In algebraic notation:

$$\begin{aligned} \text{Spec} &= d / (b + d) \\ &= d / p' \end{aligned}$$

In error notation (see Fig. 1.5):

$$\text{Spec} = (1 - \alpha)$$

In probability notation:

$$\text{Spec} = p(\text{T}- \mid \text{D}-)$$

Sens and Spec were once thought to be invariant, intrinsic test properties, independent of study sample and location. Certainly they are algebraically unrelated to the base rate, P (Sect. 1.3.2), and hence insensitive to changes in class distribution, being strict columnar ratios. However, in medical practice it is now recognised that heterogeneity of clinical populations (spectrum bias) imposes potentially serious limitations on the utility of Sens and Spec measures, since very different values may be found, for example in different patient subgroups within the sampled population, i.e. Sens and Spec are not independent of disease prevalence [3, 10, 23, 24] (Sect. 3.4).

**Worked Example: Effect of Prevalence on Sens, Spec**
In the aforementioned study of MACE [15], test performance was analysed in patient cohorts aged ≥65 years (n = 287) and ≥75 years (n = 119), in whom the prevalence of cognitive impairment (dementia and mild cognitive impairment) was anticipated to be higher than in the whole cohort, since the prevalence of dementia increases with age. The table shows Sens and Spec for cognitive impairment at the MACE cut-off of ≤25/30 (with 95% confidence intervals) in the different cohorts.

| Cohort | Whole | ≥65 years | ≥75 years |
|---|---|---|---|
| N | 755 | 287 | 119 |
| Prevalence of cognitive impairment | 0.445 | 0.749 | 0.933 |
| Sens | 0.967 (0.948–0.986) | 0.963 (0.937–0.988) | 0.991 (0.973–1.00) |
| Spec | 0.458 (0.411–0.506) | 0.528 (0.412–0.643) | 0.375 (0.040–0.710) |

Hence this analysis clearly illustrates the different values for Sens and Spec in subgroups with different disease prevalence (or pre-test probability) [18].

Sens and Spec also vary with test cut-off [15] or Q [16], prompting the development of "quality measures" (Sect. 2.2.2).

### 2.2.2 Quality Measures (QSN, QSP)

As previously discussed (Sect. 1.3.2), Kraemer [14] developed a metric, Q, the level of a test, also known as the "positive sign rate", which is the probability of a positive test in the population examined.

In literal notation (Fig. 2.1):

$$Q = (TP + FP)/N$$

In algebraic notation:

$$Q = (a+b)/N$$
$$= q/N$$

The probability of a negative test ("negative sign rate") in the population is $1 - Q$ or $Q'$.

In literal notation:

$$Q' = (FN+TN)/N$$

In algebraic notation:

$$Q' = (c+d)/N$$
$$= q'/N$$

From these values, quality sensitivity and specificity values, denoted as QSN and QSP [14], or $TPR_Q$ and $TNR_Q$, may be calculated which give the increment in each parameter beyond the level, such that:

$$QSN \text{ or } TPR_Q = (Sens-Q)/Q'$$

$$QSP \text{ or } TNR_Q = (Spec-Q')/Q$$

QSN and QSP range from 0 to 1, with higher values better, as for Sens and Spec.

---

**Worked Example: QSN, QSP**

In a screening test accuracy study of MACE [15], at the cut-off of $\leq 20/30$ (Fig. 2.2), Sens = 0.912 and Spec = 0.707 (see Sect. 2.2.1), and $Q = 0.387$ and $Q' = 0.613$ (Sect. 1.3.2) [16].

Hence the value for QSN or $TPR_Q$ is:

$$QSN = (Sens-Q)/Q'$$
$$= (0.912-0.387)/0.613$$
$$= 0.857$$

The values for QSP or $TNR_Q$ is:

$$QSP = (Spec-Q')/Q$$
$$= (0.707-0.613)/0.387$$
$$= 0.242$$

Note how these quality measures differ from Sens (lower) and Spec (very much lower).

Like Sens and Spec, QSN and QSP will vary with the chosen test cut-off. These calibrated, rescaled, or standardized indices of test parameters have been suggested to be more comparable across different samples [22]. Values of QSN and QSP are generally inferior to the corresponding values of Sens and Spec [16]. The use of these quality measures has not been widely adopted

### 2.2.3   False Positive Rate (FPR), False Negative Rate (FNR)

False positive and false negative rates denote respectively the inherent capacity or propensity of a test to detect incorrectly a condition when it is absent and not to detect it correctly when it is present. Like Sens and Spec, false positive and false negative rates are conditional probabilities with range from 0 to 1,

False positive rate or ratio (FPR) is a measure of incorrect classification. In medical practice this is the probability of the test classifying non-cases as cases, and more generally of classifying non-events as events ("overcalls"). FPR ranges from 0 to 1, with lower values better.

FPR is sometimes known as the "false alarm rate" but this latter terminology is not used here because of possible confusion with another parameter for which this term may also be used which is also known as the false discovery rate (see Sect. 2.3.3). The term "fall out" is also sometimes used to denote FPR.

In literal notation (Fig. 2.1):

$$\begin{aligned} FPR &= FP/(FP + TN) \\ &= FP/p' \end{aligned}$$

In algebraic notation:

$$\begin{aligned} FPR &= b/(b + d) \\ &= b/p' \end{aligned}$$

In error notation (see Fig. 1.5):

$$FPR = \alpha$$

In probability notation:

$$FPR = p(T+ \mid D-)$$

FPR is analogous to Type I or $\alpha$ error (Sect. 1.5). FPR is the complement, or negation, of specificity (see Sect. 3.2.2).

False negative rate or ratio (FNR), or miss rate, is another measure of incorrect classification. In medical practice it is the probability of the test classifying cases as non-cases, and more generally of classifying events or instances as non-events or non-instances ("undercalls"). FNR ranges from 0 to 1, with lower values better.

In literal notation (Fig. 2.1):

$$FNR = FN/(FN+TP)$$
$$= FN/p$$

In algebraic notation:

$$FNR = c/(a+c)$$
$$= c/p$$

In error notation (see Fig. 1.5):

$$FNR = \beta$$

In probability notation:

$$FNR = p(T-\mid D+)$$

FNR is analogous to Type II or $\beta$ error (Sect. 1.5). FNR is the complement, or negation, of sensitivity (see Sect. 3.2.1).

**Worked Example: FPR, FNR**

In a screening test accuracy study of MACE [15], at the MACE cut-off of ≤20/30, the test outcomes were as follows (Fig. 2.2): TP = 104, FN = 10, FP = 188, and TN = 453.

Hence the values for FPR and FNR at this cut-off are:

$$FPR = FP/(FP+TN)$$
$$= 188/(188+453)$$
$$= 0.293$$

$$FNR = FN/(FN+TP)$$
$$= 10/(10+104)$$
$$= 0.088$$

Like Sens and Spec, FPR and FNR are strict columnar ratios and hence algebraically are unrelated to the base rate, P, and hence are (at least notionally) insensitive to changes in class distribution. However, as with Sens and Spec, values may vary with the heterogeneity of clinical populations (spectrum bias). FPR and FNR vary with test cut-off [15].

The appropriate balance between FP and FN in any test, or their relative costs, may need to be factored into clinical judgments (see Sect. 3.2.5 for further discussion). Of note, many measures assume these costs to be equal (e.g. diagnostic odds ratio, Sect. 2.4.1; accuracy, Sect. 3.2.4; Youden index, Sect. 4.2) but this is often not the case in clinical practice.

## 2.3   Information-Based Measures

### 2.3.1   Positive and Negative Predictive Values (PPV, NPV)

Predictive values give the probability that a disease is present or absent given the test is positive or negative, or more generally that the test will forecast the correct outcome or classification [1]. Predictive values range from 0 to 1, with higher values better. Predictive values are calculated using values from both columns of the $2 \times 2$ contingency table (cf. Sens and Spec; Sect. 2.2.1), hence are sensitive to class imbalance or skews, or in other words are dependent on disease prevalence,

Positive predictive value (PPV) is the probability of disease in a patient given a positive test, also known as the post-positive test probability of disease, or post-test probability, or precision. In the weather forecasting literature, the term probability of detection (POD) or prefigurance is sometimes used [34].

In literal notation (Fig. 2.1):

$$\begin{aligned} PPV &= TP/(TP+FP) \\ &= TP/q \end{aligned}$$

In algebraic notation:

$$\begin{aligned} PPV &= a/(a+b) \\ &= a/q \end{aligned}$$

In probability notation:

$$PPV = p(D+ | T+)$$

Negative predictive value (NPV) is the probability of the absence of disease in a patient given a negative test, hence also known as the post-negative test probability of absence of disease. Hence both PPV and NPV may be described as patient-oriented measures (cf. Sens and Spec as test-oriented measures).

In literal notation (Fig. 2.1):

$$\begin{aligned} NPV &= TN/(FN+TN) \\ &= TN/q' \end{aligned}$$

In algebraic notation:

$$NPV \quad = \quad d/(c+d)$$
$$= \quad d/q'$$

In probability notation:

$$NPV \quad = \quad p(D-\mid T-)$$

---

**Worked Example: PPV, NPV**

In a screening test accuracy study of MACE [15], at the MACE cut-off of $\leq$20/30, the test outcomes were as follows (Fig. 2.2): TP = 104, FN =10, FP = 188, and TN = 453.

Hence the raw, unadjusted, predictive values at this cut-off are:

$$PPV \quad = \quad TP/(TP+FP)$$
$$= \quad 104/(104+188)$$
$$= \quad 0.356$$

$$NPV \quad = \quad TN/(FN+TN)$$
$$= \quad 453/(10+453)$$
$$= \quad 0.978$$

---

Predictive values are scalar values based on information from both columns of the 2 × 2 table (cf. Sens and Spec), hence vary with prevalence, P (Sects. 2.3.2 and 2.3.5), for which reason their values may be described as "unstable" and do not necessarily travel well from one situation to another. Predictive values also vary with the level of the test, Q, and are sensitive to class imbalance.

## 2.3.2   Bayes' Formula; Standardized Positive and Negative Predictive Values (SPPV, SNPV)

It is possible to calculate PPV and NPV at any disease prevalence based on values for Sens and Spec since the latter are (relatively) resistant to changes in prevalence, although not immutably fixed (Sect. 2.2.1). This approach to probability revision is given by Bayes' formula, after Thomas Bayes (1702-61), hence [1]:

$$PPV \quad = \quad Sens \times P/(Sens \times P)+\left[(1-Spec)\times(1-P)\right]$$
$$= \quad Sens \times P/(Sens \times P)+\left[FPR \times(1-P)\right]$$

$$\begin{aligned} \text{NPV} &= \text{Spec} \times (1-P) / \left[ \text{Spec} \times (1-P) \right] + \left[ (1-\text{Sens}) \times P \right] \\ &= \text{Spec} \times (1-P) / \left[ \text{Spec} \times (1-P) \right] + \left[ \text{FNR} \times P \right] \end{aligned}$$

This may be expressed in probability notation as:

$$\text{PPV} = p(T+\mid D+).p(D+) / p(T+\mid D+).p(D+) + p(T+\mid D-).p(D-)$$

$$\text{NPV} = p(T-\mid D-).p(D-) / p(T-\mid D-).p(D-) + p(T-\mid D+).p(D+)$$

Heston [8, 9] defined "standardized predictive values" as the predictive values calculated at 50% disease prevalence, hence:

$$\begin{aligned} \text{SPPV} &= 0.5 \times \text{Sens} / (0.5 \times \text{Sens}) + \left[ 0.5 \times (1-\text{Spec}) \right] \\ &= 0.5 \times \text{Sens} / (0.5 \times \text{Sens}) + (0.5 \times \text{FPR}) \end{aligned}$$

$$\begin{aligned} \text{SNPV} &= 0.5 \times \text{Spec} / (0.5 \times \text{Spec}) + \left[ 0.5 \times (1-\text{Sens}) \right] \\ &= 0.5 \times \text{Spec} / (0.5 \times \text{Spec}) + (0.5 \times \text{FNR}) \end{aligned}$$

Heston also suggested the potential clinical value of performing predictive value calculations for prevalence rates of 25% and 75%. Estimates of standardized predictive values, SPPV and SNPV, may differ from PPV and NPV, the differences being larger when prevalence deviates more strongly from 0.5.

**Worked Example: SPPV, SNPV**

In a screening test accuracy study of the MACE [15], at the MACE cut-off ≤20/30 (Fig. 2.2), Sens = 0.912 and Spec = 0.707 (see Sect. 2.2.1). Dementia prevalence in the patient cohort (N = 755) was 0.151 (Sect. 1.3.2).

For a dementia prevalence of 0.5, the standardized predictive values are:

$$\begin{aligned} \text{SPPV} &= 0.5 \times \text{Sens} / (0.5 \times \text{Sens}) + \left[ 0.5 \times (1-\text{Spec}) \right] \\ &= 0.5 \times 0.912 / (0.5 \times 0.912) + \left[ 0.5 \times (1-0.707) \right] \\ &= 0.757 \end{aligned}$$

$$\begin{aligned} \text{SNPV} &= 0.5 \times \text{Spec} / \left[ 0.5 \times \text{Spec} \right] + \left[ 0.5 \times (1-\text{Sens}) \right] \\ &= 0.5 \times 0.707 / \left[ 0.5 \times 0.707 \right] + \left[ 0.5 \times (1-0.912) \right] \\ &= 0.889 \end{aligned}$$

Comparing the SPPV and SNPV values with PPV and NPV (Sect. 2.3.1), SPPV is much better than PPV (0.757 vs 0.356), whilst SNPV is a little worse than NPV (0.889 vs 0.978).

This possibility for rescaling PPV and NPV for different values of P is sometimes exploited by researchers to give an indication of test performance in settings other than that of their own study. Examples amongst cognitive screening tests include the Addenbrooke's Cognitive Examination [26], the Addenbrooke's Cognitive Examination Revised [28], and the Mini-Addenbrooke's Cognitive Examination [15], with PPV and NPV calculated at prevalence rates of 0.05, 0.1, 0.2, and 0.4. PPV may be calculated across the complete range of prevalence or pretest probabilities to produce a conditional probability plot (Sect. 2.3.5).

The rescaling of Sens and Spec according to the level of the test, Q (see Sect. 2.2.2) may also be applied to other parameters. Since, from Kraemer's [14] equations:

$$QSN \quad = \quad (Sens - Q)/Q' = (NPV - P')/P$$

and

$$QSP \quad = \quad (Spec - Q')/Q = (PPV - P)/P'$$

rearranging it follows that:

$$NPV_Q \quad = \quad (QSN \times P) + P'$$

and

$$PPV_Q \quad = \quad (QSP \times P') + P$$

This allows rescaled predictive values to be calculated at different levels of Q, as for Sens and Spec being recalculated as QSN or $TPR_Q$ and QSP or $TNR_Q$ [16] (e.g. Sect. 2.2.2).

---

**Worked Examples: $PPV_Q$, $NPV_Q$**

In a screening test accuracy study of MACE [15], at the cut-off $\leq 20/30$, QSN = 0.857 and QSP = 0.242 (see Sect. 2.2.2), and dementia prevalence in the patient cohort (N = 755) was P = 0.151 (Sect. 1.3.2).

Hence the values for $PPV_Q$ and $NPV_Q$ are:

$$
\begin{aligned}
PPV_Q \quad &= \quad (QSP \times P') + P \\
&= \quad (0.242 \times 0.849) + 0.151 \\
&= \quad 0.356
\end{aligned}
$$

$$
\begin{aligned}
NPV_Q \quad &= \quad (QSN \times P) + P' \\
&= \quad (0.857 \times 0.151) + 0.849 \\
&= \quad 0.978
\end{aligned}
$$

These values are identical to the unscaled values of PPV and NPV (Sect. 2.3.1) because the same MACE cut-off was used, hence the positive sign rate $Q = 0.387$ (Sect. 1.3.2) was the same. If we select a different value of Q, say 0.5, then:

$$
\begin{aligned}
\text{QSN} &= (\text{Sens} - Q)/Q' \\
&= (0.912 - 0.5)/0.5 \\
&= 0.824
\end{aligned}
$$

$$
\begin{aligned}
\text{QSP} &= (\text{Spec} - Q')/Q \\
&= (0.707 - 0.5)/0.5 \\
&= 0.414
\end{aligned}
$$

Hence the values for $\text{PPV}_Q$ and $\text{NPV}_Q$ are now:

$$
\begin{aligned}
\text{PPV}_Q &= (\text{QSP} \times P') + P \\
&= (0.414 \times 0.849) + 0.151 \\
&= 0.502
\end{aligned}
$$

$$
\begin{aligned}
\text{NPV}_Q &= (\text{QSN} \times P) + P' \\
&= (0.824 \times 0.151) + 0.849 \\
&= 0.973
\end{aligned}
$$

With the change in Q, QSN and particularly $\text{NPV}_Q$ have changed little, reflecting the high sensitivity of MACE, whereas QSP and $\text{PPV}_Q$ have shown greater change.

## 2.3.3 False Discovery Rate (FDR), False Reassurance Rate (FRR)

The false discovery rate (FDR) is a measure of the probability of the absence of disease given an abnormal test (i.e. identifying a non-case as a case), hence also known as the post-positive test probability of absence of disease. FDR ranges from 0 to 1, with lower values better.

FDR has sometimes been known as the false alarm rate. "False alarm rate" is potentially an ambiguous term: it has also been used on occasion to mean both the false positive rate (FPR) (e.g. [14], p.64] and the false negative rate (FNR) [32] (Sect. 2.2.3). Hence the FDR terminology is preferred here in order to avoid any possible confusion.

In literal notation (Fig. 2.1):

$$FDR = FP/(TP+FP)$$
$$= FP/q$$

In algebraic notation:

$$FDR = b/(a+b)$$
$$= b/q$$

FDR is the complement of PPV (see Sect. 3.3.1):

$$FDR = 1-PPV$$

In probability notation:

$$FDR = p(D-\mid T+)$$

By Bayes' equation:

$$FDR = p(T+\mid D-).p(D-)/p(T+\mid D-).p(D-)+p(T+\mid D+).p(D+)$$

False reassurance rate (FRR), sometimes known as false omission rate (FOR), is a measure of the probability of the presence of disease given a normal test (i.e. identifying a case as a non-case), hence also known as the post-negative test probability of disease. FRR ranges from 0 to 1, with lower values better.
In literal notation (Fig. 2.1):

$$FRR = FN/(FN+TN)$$
$$= FN/q'$$

In algebraic notation:

$$FRR = c/(c+d)$$
$$= c/q'$$

FRR is the complement of NPV (see Sect. 3.3.2):

$$FRR = 1-NPV$$

In probability notation:

$$FRR = p(D+\mid T-)$$

By Bayes' equation:

$$FRR = p(T-\mid D+).p(D+)/p(T-\mid D+).p(D+)+p(T-\mid D-).p(D-)$$

**Worked Example: FDR, FRR**

In a screening test accuracy study of MACE [15], at the MACE cut-off of $\leq 20/30$ (Fig. 2.2), TP = 104, FN = 10, FP = 188, and TN = 453.

Hence the values for FDR and FRR are:

$$
\begin{aligned}
\text{FDR} &= \text{FP}/(\text{TP}+\text{FP}) \\
&= 188/(104+188) \\
&= 0.644
\end{aligned}
$$

$$
\begin{aligned}
\text{FRR} &= \text{FN}/(\text{FN}+\text{TN}) \\
&= 10/(10+453) \\
&= 0.0215
\end{aligned}
$$

### 2.3.4   Positive and Negative Likelihood Ratios (LR+, LR−)

Likelihood ratios (LRs), also sometimes known as diagnostic likelihood ratios (DLRs), measure the change in pre-test odds (Sect. 1.3.3) to post-test odds (Sect. 2.3.5), and hence may be characterised as measures of probability revision based on Bayes' formula, or measures of diagnostic gain. They combine information about sensitivity and specificity [32] and hence are closely related to these terms.

The positive likelihood ratio (LR+, also sometimes denoted PLR) gives the odds of a positive test result in an affected individual relative to an unaffected:

$$
\begin{aligned}
\text{LR+} &= \text{Sens}/(1-\text{Spec}) \\
&= \text{Sens}/\text{FPR} \\
&= \text{TPR}/\text{FPR}
\end{aligned}
$$

In literal notation:

$$
\begin{aligned}
\text{LR+} &= \left[\text{TP}/(\text{TP}+\text{FN})\right]/\left[\text{FP}/(\text{FP}+\text{TN})\right] \\
&= \left[\text{TP}/\text{p}\right]/\left[\text{FP}/\text{p}'\right] \\
&= \left[\text{TP}.\text{p}'\right]/\left[\text{FP}.\text{p}\right]
\end{aligned}
$$

In algebraic notation:

$$
\begin{aligned}
\text{LR+} &= \left[\text{a}/(\text{a}+\text{c})\right]/\left[\text{b}/(\text{b}+\text{d})\right] \\
&= \left[\text{a}.(\text{b}+\text{d})\right]/\left[\text{b}.(\text{a}+\text{c})\right] \\
&= \left[\text{a}.\text{p}'\right]/\left[\text{b}.\text{p}\right]
\end{aligned}
$$

In error notation:

$$LR+ \quad = \quad (1-\beta)/\alpha$$

LR+ can also be expressed in probability notation:

$$LR+ \quad = \quad TPR / FPR$$
$$= \quad p(T+ \mid D+)/ p(T+ \mid D-)$$

If the outcome of a test is $R_i$, then more generally:

$$LR \quad = \quad p(R_i \mid D+)/ p(R_i \mid D-)$$

The negative likelihood ratio (LR−, also sometimes denoted NLR) gives the odds of a negative test result in an affected individual relative to an unaffected.

$$LR- \quad = \quad (1-Sens)/Spec$$
$$= \quad FNR / Spec$$
$$= \quad FNR / TNR$$

In literal notation:

$$LR- \quad = \quad \left[ FN/(TP+FN) \right]/\left[ TN/(FP+TN) \right]$$
$$= \quad \left[ FN/p \right]/\left[ TN/p' \right]$$
$$= \quad \left[ FN.p' \right]/\left[ TN.p \right]$$

In algebraic notation:

$$LR- \quad = \quad \left[ c/(a+c) \right]/\left[ d/(b+d) \right]$$
$$= \quad \left[ c.(b+d) \right]/\left[ d.(a+c) \right]$$
$$= \quad \left[ c.p' \right]/\left[ d.p \right]$$

In error notation:

$$LR- \quad = \quad \beta/(1-\alpha)$$

LR− can also be expressed in probability notation:

$$LR- \quad = \quad FNR / TNR$$
$$= \quad p(T- \mid D+)/ p(T- \mid D-)$$

Likelihood ratios may be qualitatively classified according to their distance from 1, a useless test, to indicate the change in probability of disease (Table 2.1, left hand column) [13]; for LR+ end points are 1 to ∞; for LR− they are 0 to 1.

**Table 2.1**  Classification of LRs

| LR value | Qualitative classification: Change in probability of disease [12] | Approximate change in probability (%) [27] |
|---|---|---|
| ≤ 0.1 | Very large decrease | – |
| 0.1 | Large decrease | –45 |
| ≤ 0.2 | Large decrease | –30 |
| 0.3 | Moderate decrease | –25 |
| 0.4 | Moderate decrease | –20 |
| ≤ 0.5 | Moderate decrease | –15 |
| 0.5 < LR− ≤ 1.0 | Slight decrease | – |
| 1.0 | | 0 |
| 1.0 < LR+ < 2.0 | Slight increase | – |
| 2.0 | Moderate increase | +15 |
| 3.0 | Moderate increase | +20 |
| 4.0 | Moderate increase | +25 |
| ≤ 5.0 | Moderate increase | +30 |
| 6.0 | Large increase | +35 |
| 8.0 | Large increase | +40 |
| ≤ 10.0 | Large increase | +45 |
| ≥ 10.0 | Very large increase | – |

A distinction may be drawn between result-specific and category-specific LRs ([12], p.175). A result-specific LR refers to the ratio of the probability of observing that result conditional on the presence of the target (disease, diagnosis) to the probability of observing that result conditional on the absence of the target. More often in clinical practice dichotomised test results are cumulated to produce a category-specific LR.

> **Worked Example: Result-Specific LR**
> The "attended with" (AW) sign has been proposed as a useful screening test for the diagnosis of cognitive impairment. In a screening test accuracy study in a large consecutive patient cohort (N = 1209), AW sign was observed in 473 of 507 patients with major and minor neurocognitive disorder and in 306 of 702 patients with no cognitive impairment [19].
> Hence, the probability of AW given cognitive impairment is 473/507 = 0.933, and the probability of AW given no cognitive impairment is 306/702 = 0.436. Note that these values are equivalent to the true positive rate (TPR) or

sensitivity of the test and the false positive rate (FPR). Hence the result-specific likelihood ratio is given by:

$$
\begin{aligned}
LR &= p(R_i \mid D+)/p(R_i \mid D-) \\
&= TPR / FPR \\
&= 0.933 / 0.436 \\
&= 2.14
\end{aligned}
$$

Following the qualitative classification of likelihood ratios described by Jaeschke et al. [13], LR = 2.14 represents a moderate increase in the probability of disease.

**Worked Example: Category-Specific LR+, LR−**

In a screening test accuracy study of the MACE [15], at the MACE cut-off ≤20/30, Sens = 0.912 and Spec = 0.707 for dementia diagnosis (Sect. 2.2.1). Hence, the positive likelihood ratio (LR+) at this cut-off is:

$$
\begin{aligned}
LR+ &= Sens /(1-Spec) \\
&= 0.912 /(1-0.707) \\
&= 3.11
\end{aligned}
$$

Following the qualitative classification of likelihood ratios described by Jaeschke et al. [13], LR+ = 3.11 represents a moderate increase in the probability of disease.

The negative likelihood ratio (LR−) at this cut-off is:

$$
\begin{aligned}
LR- &= (1-Sens)/Spec \\
&= (1-0.912)/0.707 \\
&= 0.124
\end{aligned}
$$

Following the qualitative classification of likelihood ratios described by Jaeschke et al. [13], LR− = 0.124 represents a large decrease in the probability of disease.

Note that these results could also be obtained from the raw study data (see Fig. 2.2). For LR+, the probability of MACE ≤20/30 given dementia is 104/114 = 0.912 (equivalent to sensitivity or true positive rate) and the probability of MACE ≤20/30 given no dementia is 188/641 = 0.293

(equivalent to false positive rate; Sect. 2.2.3). Hence the category-specific positive likelihood ratio is given by:

$$LR+ = p(T+|D+)/p(T+|D-)$$
$$= TPR/FPR$$
$$= 0.912/0.293$$
$$= 3.11$$

For LR−, the probability of MACE >20/30 given dementia is 10/114 = 0.088 (equivalent to false negative rate; Sect. 2.2.3) and the probability of MACE >20/30 given no dementia is 453/641 = 0.707 (equivalent to specificity or true negative rate). Hence the category-specific negative likelihood ratio is given by:

$$LR- = p(T-|D+)/p(T-|D-)$$
$$= FNR/TNR$$
$$= 0.088/0.707$$
$$= 0.124$$

As LRs are derived from sensitivity and specificity, like these metrics they are algebraically unrelated to the base rate, P. However, as is the case for Sens and Spec, in practice LRs are not independent of prevalence [3].

LRs vary with test cut-off [15] (see also Fig. 7.2). Rather than dichotomising outcomes with a single cut-off, dividing continuous data into intervals and calculating interval likelihood ratios (ILRs) is possible [4] (Sect. 7.3.2).

LRs may be rescaled according to the level of the test, Q (see Sect. 2.2.2) [16], such that:

$$LR_Q+ = QSN/(1-QSP)$$

$$LR_Q- = (1-QSN)/QSP$$

Calculation of LRs also provides a method for combining the results of multiple tests, assuming conditional independence of the tests in the presence and absence of the target diagnosis:

$$Post\text{-}test\ odds = Pre\text{-}test\ odds \times LR_1 \times LR_2 + \ldots LR_n$$

Combination of test results is further considered in Section 7.3.4.

## 2.3.5   Post-test Odds; Net Harm to Net Benefit (H/B) Ratio

Post-test odds may be calculated as the product of LR+ and the pre-test odds (Sect. 1.3.2), a form of Bayesian updating:

$$\text{Post-test odds} = \text{Pre-test odds} \times \text{LR+}$$
$$= (P/P') \times \text{LR+}$$

In probability notation:

$$\text{Post-test odds} = p(D+)/p(D-) \times \text{LR+}$$

---

**Worked Example: Post-test Odds**
In the screening test accuracy study of MACE [15], the pre-test odds of dementia were 0.178 (Sect. 1.3.2). The positive likelihood ratio, LR+, of MACE using the cut-off ≤20/30 was 3.11 (Sect. 2.3.4).
Hence the post-test odds of dementia using MACE cut-off ≤20/30 are:

$$\text{Post-test odds} = \text{Pre-test odds} \times \text{LR+}$$
$$= 0.178 \times 3.11$$
$$= 0.553$$

If desired, post-test odds may be converted back to a post-test probability, for comparison with the pre-test probability:

$$\text{Post-test probability} = \text{Post-test odds}/(1 + \text{post-test odds})$$
$$= 0.553/1.553$$
$$= 0.356$$

This may be compared with the pre-test probability in this cohort of 0.151 (Sect. 1.3.2), indicating the added value of the test.

---

McGee [27] advocated some simple rules to obviate these calculations between pre- and post-test odds and probabilities, such that LR+ values of 2, 5, and 10 increased the probability by 15%, 30%, and 45% respectively, whereas LR− values of 0.5, 0.2, and 0.1 decreased the probability by 15%, 30% and 45% respectively (Table 2.1, right hand column). These approximate figures derive from the almost linear relationship of probability and the natural logarithm of odds over the range 10% to 90%, such that the change in probability may be calculated independent of pre-test probability:

$$\text{Change in probability} = 0.19 \times \log_e(\text{LR})$$

The post-test odds may also be characterised as the ratio of net harm to net benefit (H/B), that is the harm (H) of treating a person without disease (i.e. a false positive) to the net benefit (B) of treating a person with disease (i.e. a true positive), the latter term equating to the harm of a false negative result [7]. H/B ratio may also be calculated using Bayes' equation:

$$\text{Net Harm}(H) / \text{Net Benefit}(B) = \text{Pre-test odds} \times \text{LR}+$$
$$= (P / P') \times \text{LR}+$$
$$= (P / P') \times (\text{TPR} / \text{FPR})$$

For the net harm to net benefit (H/B) ratio, higher values are desirable if the harm of a false negative (missing a case) is deemed more significant than the harm of diagnosing a false positive (identifying a non-case as a case), a view most clinicians would hold to (Sect. 3.2.5). A higher H/B ratio means the test is less likely to miss cases, and hence less likely to incur the harms of false negatives. (This scoring of H/B ratio may seem counterintuitive if one thinks solely of "harms" and "benefits", hence the important qualification of "net"). Tests with high sensitivity may nevertheless have an undesirably low H/B ratio if they also have poor specificity [20].

This equation is also pertinent to considerations of misclassification cost (Sect. 3.2.5) as harms are sometimes characterised as "costs" and hence the term cost:benefit ratio is sometimes used. Also, since TPR/FPR is equivalent to the slope of the receiver operating characteristic (ROC) curve ([12], p.68, 157, 171), this is also relevant to the setting of test cut-offs using the ROC curve (Section 6.2).

## 2.3.6   Conditional Probability Plot

A conditional probability plot may be used to illustrate graphically the variation in post-test probability across the complete range of pre-test probabilities (Fig. 2.3). Two curves are generated: one for $p(D+ \mid T+)$, or PPV; and one for $p(D+ \mid T-)$, or FRR (Table 2.2, left hand columns). The point at $P = 0.5$ on the test-positive plot corresponds to the standardized positive predictive value (SPPV; Sect. 2.3.2) and at $P = 0.5$ on the test-negative plot corresponds to $(1 - \text{SNPV})$. The diagonal line corresponds to the situation where a test has LR+ = 1, such that pre-test and post-test probabilities are equal and the test result contributes no information.

Clearly, the shape of the conditional probability plot is dependent on the chosen test cut-off (i.e. Q). For example, contrast the plots for MACE cut-off $\leq 20/30$ (Fig. 2.3) with cut-off $\leq 25/30$ (from the index study [10]; Fig. 2.4 and Table 2.2, right hand columns). With the higher cut-off, the test-negative plot is further from the LR = 1 diagonal than with the lower cut-off, indicating that $p(D+ \mid T-)$ is extremely low at this test threshold, suggesting this it is very good for ruling out disease (few false negatives, high NPV). The test-positive line is closer to LR = 1, indicating that $p(D+ \mid T+)$ at this threshold is not as effective as the lower threshold

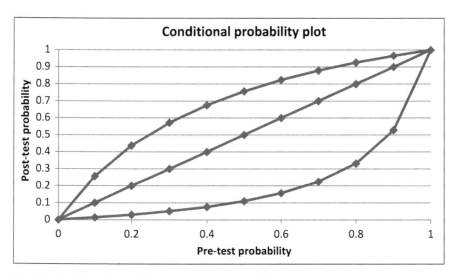

**Fig. 2.3** Conditional probability plot of post-test probability (dependent variable; y axis) vs pre-test probability (independent variable; x axis) of MACE for dementia diagnosis at cut-off ≤20/30 (data from [21], p.157). Upper curve (test positive) corresponds to PPV (see Fig. 3.10); lower curve (test negative) corresponds to FRR (see Fig. 3.11).

**Table 2.2** Values of PPV and FRR for dementia diagnosis at fixed MACE cut-offs of ≤20/30 (left) and ≤25/30 (right) at various prevalence levels, correspondingly to Figs. 2.3 and 2.4 respectively

| P, P′ | MACE cut-off ≤20/30 | | MACE cut-off ≤25/30 | |
|---|---|---|---|---|
|  | PPV | FRR | PPV | FRR |
| 0.1, 0.9 | 0.257 | 0.014 | 0.138 | 0.003 |
| 0.2, 0.8 | 0.437 | 0.030 | 0.266 | 0.007 |
| 0.3, 0.7 | 0.571 | 0.051 | 0.383 | 0.012 |
| 0.4, 0.6 | 0.675 | 0.076 | 0.491 | 0.019 |
| 0.5, 0.5 | 0.757 | 0.110 | 0.591 | 0.028 |
| 0.6, 0.4 | 0.824 | 0.157 | 0.685 | 0.041 |
| 0.7, 0.3 | 0.879 | 0.225 | 0.771 | 0.063 |
| 0.8, 0.2 | 0.926 | 0.332 | 0.853 | 0.103 |
| 0.9, 0.1 | 0.966 | 0.528 | 0.929 | 0.205 |

for ruling disease in (lower LR+). Dependence of test parameters on Q is considered further in the next chapter.

## 2.3.7  *Positive and Negative Predictive Ratios (PPR, NPR)*

Linn described two measures which are analogous to likelihood ratios (Sect. 2.3.4) but based on predictive values (Sect. 2.3.1) rather than Sens and Spec (Sect. 2.2.1), and named predictive ratios [25].

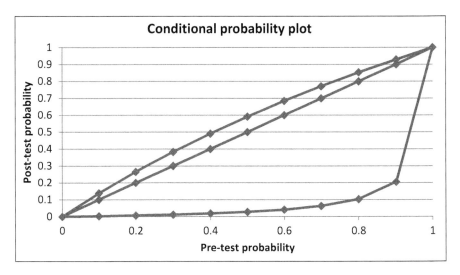

**Fig. 2.4** Conditional probability plot of post-test probability vs pre-test probability of MACE for dementia diagnosis at cut-off ≤25/30. Compare with Fig. 2.3

The positive predictive ratio (PPR) is given by:

$$PPR = PPV/(1-NPV)$$
$$= PPV/FRR$$

In literal notation:

$$PPR = \left[TP/(TP+FP)\right]/\left[FN/(FN+TN)\right]$$
$$= \left[TP/q\right]/\left[FN/q'\right]$$
$$= \left[TP.q'\right]/\left[FN.q\right]$$

In algebraic notation:

$$PPR = \left[a/(a+b)\right]/\left[c/(c+d)\right]$$
$$= \left[a.(c+d)\right]/\left[c.(a+b)\right]$$
$$= \left[a.q'\right]/\left[c.q\right]$$

In probability notation:

$$PPR = p(D+\mid T+)/p(D+\mid T-)$$

By Bayes' equation:

$$PPR = \left[p(T+\mid D+).p(D+)/p(T+\mid D+).p(D+)+p(T+\mid D-).p(D-)\right] \div$$
$$\left[p(T-\mid D+).p(D+)/p(T-\mid D+).p(D+)+p(T-\mid D-).p(D-)\right]$$

The negative predictive ratio (NPR) is given by:

$$NPR = (1 - PPV)/NPV$$
$$= FDR/NPV$$

In literal notation:

$$NPR = \left[FP/(TP+FP)\right]/\left[TN/(FN+TN)\right]$$
$$= \left[FP/q\right]/\left[TN/q'\right]$$
$$= \left[FP.q'\right]/\left[TN.q\right]$$

In algebraic notation:

$$NPR = \left[b/(a+b)\right]/\left[d/(c+d)\right]$$
$$= \left[b.(c+d)\right]/\left[d.(a+b)\right]$$
$$= \left[b.q'\right]/\left[d.q\right]$$

In probability notation:

$$NPR = p(D-\mid T+)/p(D-\mid T-)$$

By Bayes' equation:

$$NPR = [p(T+\mid D-)\,p(D-)/p(T+\mid D-)\,p(D-)+p(T+\mid D+)\,p(D+)] \div p(T-\mid D-)\,p(D-)/p(T-\mid D-)\,p(D-)+p(T-\mid D+)\,p(D+)$$

---

**Worked Example: PPR, NPR**

In a screening test accuracy study of the MACE [15], at the MACE cut-off ≤20/30, PPV = 0.356 and NPV = 0.978 (Sect. 2.3.1).

Hence, the positive predictive ratio (PPR) at this cut-off is:

$$PPR = PPV/(1-NPV)$$
$$= 0.356/(1-0.978)$$
$$= 0.356/0.02159$$
$$= 16.49$$

The negative predictive ratio (NPR) is:

$$NPR = (1-PPV)/NPV$$
$$= (1-0.356)/0.978$$
$$= 0.658$$

As for LRs, these results can also be obtained from the raw study data (see Fig. 2.2). For PPR, the probability of dementia given MACE ≤20/30 is 104/292 = 0.356 (equivalent to positive predictive value) and the probability of dementia given MACE >20/30 is 10/463 = 0.022 (equivalent to false reassurance rate; Sect. 2.3.3). Hence PPR is given by:

$$
\begin{aligned}
\text{PPR} \ &= \ p\!\left(\text{D}+\mid \text{T}+\right)/\,p\!\left(\text{D}+\mid \text{T}-\right) \\
&= \ \text{PPV}/\text{FRR} \\
&= \ 0.356/0.02159 \\
&= \ 16.49
\end{aligned}
$$

For NPR, the probability of no dementia given MACE ≤20/30 is 188/292 = 0.644 (equivalent to false discovery rate; Sect. 2.3.3) and the probability of no dementia given MACE >20/30 is 453/463 = 0.978 (equivalent to negative predictive value). Hence NPR is given by:

$$
\begin{aligned}
\text{NPR} \ &= \ p\!\left(\text{D}-\mid \text{T}+\right)/\,p\!\left(\text{D}-\mid \text{T}-\right) \\
&= \ \text{FDR}/\text{NPV} \\
&= \ 0.644/0.978 \\
&= \ 0.658
\end{aligned}
$$

PPR and NPR values are seldom examined in practice [2].


## 2.4   Association-Based Measures

### 2.4.1   Diagnostic Odds Ratio (DOR) and Error Odds Ratio (EOR)

The diagnostic odds ratio (DOR) or the cross product ratio [5, 6] is the ratio of the product of true positives and true negatives and of false negatives and false positives.
In literal notation:

$$
\text{DOR} \ = \ \left(\text{TP}\times\text{TN}\right)/\left(\text{FP}\times\text{FN}\right)
$$

In algebraic notation:

$$
\text{DOR} \ = \ \left(\text{ad}\right)/\left(\text{bc}\right)
$$

DOR may also be expressed in terms of other previously encountered parameters (Sens, Spec, likelihood ratios, predictive values, and predictive ratios):

$$
\begin{aligned}
\text{DOR} &= (\text{Sens} \times \text{Spec}) / [(1 - \text{Sens}) \times (1 - \text{Spec})] \\
&= (\text{Sens} \times \text{Spec}) / (\text{FNR} \times \text{FPR}) \\
&= (\text{TPR} \times \text{TNR}) / (\text{FNR} \times \text{FPR}) \\
&= [\text{TPR} / (1 - \text{TPR})] \times [(1 - \text{FPR}) / \text{FPR}] \\
&= \text{LR+} / \text{LR-} \\
&= \text{PPV} \times \text{NPV} / (1 - \text{PPV}) \times (1 - \text{NPV}) \\
&= \text{PPV} \times \text{NPV} / \text{FDR} \times \text{FRR} \\
&= \text{PPR} / \text{NPR}
\end{aligned}
$$

Hence, from LRs, in error notation:

$$
\begin{aligned}
\text{DOR} &= [(1 - \beta) / \alpha] / [\beta / (1 - \alpha)] \\
&= (1 - \beta)(1 - \alpha) / (\alpha \beta)
\end{aligned}
$$

DOR may range from 1, a random classifier (useless test), to +/- ∞ if any of the cells of the 2 × 2 table is zero, hence there are no fixed end points. A rescaling to a weighted kappa statistic with endpoints of 0 (random classifier) and 1 (perfect classifier) has been described [35]. A qualitative classification of DOR values was suggested by Rosenthal, as: small ~1.5, medium ~2.5, large ~4, and very large ~10 or greater [33].

DOR has known shortcomings [14, 17]. It treats FN and FP as equally undesirable, which is often not the case in clinical practice (see Sect. 3.2.5). By choosing

---

**Worked Examples: DOR**

In a screening test accuracy study of MACE [15], at the MACE cut-off of ≤20/30 (Fig. 2.2), TP = 104, FN = 10, FP = 188, and TN = 453.

Hence the value for DOR at this cut-off is:

$$
\begin{aligned}
\text{DOR} &= (\text{TP} \times \text{TN}) / (\text{FP} \times \text{FN}) \\
&= 104 \times 453 / 188 \times 10 \\
&= 25.06
\end{aligned}
$$

Knowing Sens (0.912) and Spec (0.707) at this cut-off (Sect. 2.2.1), DOR could also be calculated thus:

$$
\begin{aligned}
\text{DOR} &= (\text{Sens} \times \text{Spec}) / [(1 - \text{Sens}) \times (1 - \text{Spec})] \\
&= 0.912 \times 0.707 / (1 - 0.912) \times (1 - 0.707) \\
&= 0.645 / 0.088 \times 0.293 \\
&= 25.01
\end{aligned}
$$

Knowing LR+ (3.11) and LR− (0.124) at this cut-off (Sect. 2.3.4), DOR could also be calculated thus:

$$
\begin{aligned}
\text{DOR} &= \text{LR+/LR−} \\
&= 3.11/0.124 \\
&= 25.08
\end{aligned}
$$

Knowing PPR (16.49) and NPR (0.658) at this cut-off (Sect. 2.3.7), DOR could also be calculated thus:

$$
\begin{aligned}
\text{DOR} &= \text{PPR/NPR} \\
&= 16.49/0.658 \\
&= 25.06
\end{aligned}
$$

[The slight differences in results relate to rounding errors.]
Following the qualitative classification of DORs described by Rosenthal [33], DOR >25 represents a very large value.

the best quality of a test and ignoring its weaknesses, it gives the most optimistic results, particularly in populations with very high or very low risk. Ratios become unstable and inflated as the denominator approaches zero, and may be zero or infinite if one of the classes is nil.

As small differences in one cell value can drastically alter DOR, use of the logarithm of the DOR is sometimes used to compensate. As DOR is a combination of products and quotients this is easily done (either common or natural logs may be used):

$$
\begin{aligned}
\log(\text{DOR}) &= \log(\text{TP})+\log(\text{TN})-\log(\text{FP})-\log(\text{FN}) \\
&= \log(a)+\log(d)-\log(b)-\log(c)
\end{aligned}
$$

log(DOR) may also be calculated from Sens and Spec, specifically from their logits (logarithms of odds):

$$
\begin{aligned}
\text{DOR} &= (\text{Sens}\times\text{Spec})/\left[(1-\text{Sens})\times(1-\text{Spec})\right] \\
\log(\text{DOR}) &= \log\left[\text{Sens}/(1-\text{Sens})\right]+\log\left[\text{Spec}/(1-\text{Spec})\right] \\
&= \text{logit}(\text{Sens})+\text{logit}(\text{Spec})
\end{aligned}
$$

**Worked Example: Log(DOR)**

In a screening test accuracy study of MACE [15], at the MACE cut-off of ≤20/30, Sens = 0.912 and Spec = 0.707 (Sect. 2.2.1).

Hence the value for log(DOR) at this cut-off, using common logs, is:

$$
\begin{aligned}
\log(DOR) &= \log\big[\text{Sens}/(1-\text{Sens})\big] + \log\big[\text{Spec}/(1-\text{Spec})\big] \\
&= \log[0.912/0.088] + \log[0.707/0.293] \\
&= 1.0155 + 0.38255 \\
&= 1.3981 \\
\text{Antilog} \quad &= DOR = 25.01
\end{aligned}
$$

$Log_e(DOR)$ is used as an accuracy parameter in meta-analysis when model fitting summary ROC curves.

The relation of DOR to Sens and Spec may also be seen graphically in the receiver operating characteristic (ROC) plot (Sect. 6.2), and of log(DOR) to log likelihood ratios in the ROC plot in likelihood ratio coordinates (Sect. 6.3.1).

As DOR is related to cut-off and hence Q, a rescaled DOR may also be calculated [16]:

$$
DOR_Q \quad = \quad LR_Q^{+}/LR_Q^{-}
$$

An error odds ratio (EOR) may also be defined, as the ratio of the product of true positives and false positives and of true negatives and false negatives.

In literal notation:

$$
EOR \quad = \quad (TP \times FP)/(FN \times TN)
$$

In algebraic notation:

$$
EOR \quad = \quad (ab)/(cd)
$$

EOR is seldom examined and not recommended [2].

**Worked Example: EOR**

In a screening test accuracy study of MACE [15], at the MACE cut-off of ≤20/30 (Fig. 2.2), TP = 104, FN =10, FP = 188, and TN = 453.

Hence the values for EOR at this cut-off is:

$$
\begin{aligned}
EOR &= (TP \times FP)/(FN \times TN) \\
&= 104 \times 188 / 10 \times 453 \\
&= 4.32
\end{aligned}
$$

## 2.4.2  *Clinical Utility Index (CUI+, CUI−) and Clinical Disutility Index (CDI+, CDI−)*

The clinical utility indexes developed by Mitchell [29] calculate the value of a diagnostic method for ruling in or ruling out a diagnosis.

Positive clinical utility index (CUI+) is given by:

$$\begin{aligned} \text{CUI+} &= \text{Sens} \times \text{PPV} \\ &= \text{TPR} \times \text{PPV} \end{aligned}$$

In literal notation:

$$\begin{aligned} \text{CUI+} &= \text{TP}/(\text{TP}+\text{FN}) \times \text{TP}/(\text{TP}+\text{FP}) \\ &= \text{TP}^2/\left[(\text{TP}+\text{FN}).(\text{TP}+\text{FP})\right] \\ &= \text{TP}^2/[\text{p}.\text{q}] \end{aligned}$$

In algebraic notation:

$$\begin{aligned} \text{CUI+} &= a/(a+c) \times a/(a+b) \\ &= a^2/\left[(a+c).(a+b)\right] \\ &= a^2/[\text{p}.\text{q}] \end{aligned}$$

This parameter has also been termed the Screening Marker Index [31].

Negative clinical utility index (CUI−) is given by:

$$\begin{aligned} \text{CUI−} &= \text{Spec} \times \text{NPV} \\ &= \text{TNR} \times \text{NPV} \end{aligned}$$

In literal notation:

$$\begin{aligned} \text{CUI−} &= \text{TN}/(\text{FP}+\text{TN}) \times \text{TN}/(\text{FN}+\text{TN}) \\ &= \text{TN}^2/\left[(\text{FP}+\text{TN}).(\text{FN}+\text{TN})\right] \\ &= \text{TN}^2/[\text{p}'.\text{q}'] \end{aligned}$$

In algebraic notation:

$$\begin{aligned} \text{CUI−} &= d/(b+d) \times d/(c+d) \\ &= d^2/\left[(b+d).(c+d)\right] \\ &= d^2/[\text{p}'.\text{q}'] \end{aligned}$$

Clinical utility index values range from 0 to 1, with higher values better. In addition to the absolute score, the qualitative performance of CUI values may be classified as: excellent ≥0.81, good ≥0.64, adequate ≥0.49, poor ≥0.36, or very poor <0.36 [29].

**Worked Example: CUI+, CUI−**
In a screening test accuracy study of the MACE [15], at the MACE cut-off of ≤20/30, Sens = 0.912 and Spec = 0.707 (Sect. 2.2.1), and PPV = 0.356 and NPV = 0.978 (Sect. 2.3.1).
   Hence, the positive clinical utility index (CUI+) at this cut-off is:

$$
\begin{aligned}
\text{CUI+} &= \text{Sens} \times \text{PPV} \\
&= 0.912 \times 0.356 \\
&= 0.325
\end{aligned}
$$

Following the qualitative classification of clinical utility indexes described by Mitchell [29], CUI+ = 0.325 is very poor.
   The negative clinical utility index (CUI−) is:

$$
\begin{aligned}
\text{CUI−} &= \text{Spec} \times \text{NPV} \\
&= 0.707 \times 0.978 \\
&= 0.691
\end{aligned}
$$

Following the qualitative classification of clinical utility indexes described by Mitchell [29], CUI− = 0.691 is good.

Rescaled CUIs may also be calculated [16]:

$$
\text{CUI}_Q+ = \text{QSN} \times \text{PPV}
$$

$$
\text{CUI}_Q− = \text{QSP} \times \text{NPV}
$$

Clinical disutility indexes (CDI) may also be developed, to calculate the limitation of a diagnostic method for ruling in or ruling out a diagnosis, such that:

$$
\begin{aligned}
\text{CDI+} &= (1 - \text{Sens}) \times (1 - \text{PPV}) \\
&= \text{FNR} \times \text{FDR}
\end{aligned}
$$

This is a measure of incorrectly ruling out.

$$
\begin{aligned}
\text{CDI−} &= (1 - \text{Spec}) \times (1 - \text{NPV}) \\
&= \text{FPR} \times \text{FRR}
\end{aligned}
$$

This is a measure of incorrectly ruling in.
   As for CUI, clinical disutility index values range from 0 to 1, but with lower values better. In addition to the absolute score, the qualitative performance of CDI

might be classified, after CUI, as: very poor $\geq$0.81, poor $\geq$0.64, adequate $\geq$0.49, good $\geq$0.36, or excellent <0.36.

---

**Worked Example: CDI+, CDI−**

In a screening test accuracy study of the MACE [15], at the MACE cut-off of $\leq$20/30, Sens = 0.912 and Spec = 0.707 (Sect. 2.2.1), and PPV = 0.356 and NPV = 0.978 (Sect. 2.3.1). Hence FNR = 0.088 and FPR = 0.293 (Sect. 2.2.3) and FDR = 0.644 and FRR = 0.022 (Sect. 2.3.3).

Hence, the positive clinical disutility index (CDI+) at this cut-off is:

$$
\begin{aligned}
CDI+ &= FNR \times FDR \\
&= 0.088 \times 0.644 \\
&= 0.057
\end{aligned}
$$

Following the suggested qualitative classification of clinical disutility indexes, CDI+ = 0.057 is excellent, suggesting the test is unlikely to rule out the diagnosis incorrectly.

The negative clinical disutility index (CDI−) is:

$$
\begin{aligned}
CDI- &= FPR \times FRR \\
&= 0.293 \times 0.022 \\
&= 0.006
\end{aligned}
$$

Following the suggested qualitative classification of clinical disutility indexes, CDI− = 0.006 is excellent, suggesting the test is unlikely to rule in the diagnosis incorrectly.

---

# References

1. Altman DG, Bland JM. Diagnostic tests 2: predictive values. BMJ. 1994;309:102.
2. Bossuyt PMM. Clinical validity: defining biomarker performance. Scand J Clin Lab Invest. 2010;70(Suppl242):46–52.
3. Brenner H, Gefeller O. Variation of sensitivity, specificity, likelihood ratios and predictive values with disease prevalence. Stat Med. 1997;16:981–91.
4. Brown MD, Reeves MJ. Interval likelihood ratios: another advantage for the evidence-based diagnostician. Ann Emerg Med. 2003;42:292–7.
5. Edwards AWF. The measure of association in a 2 × 2 table. J R Stat Soc Ser A. 1963;126:109–14.
6. Glas AS, Lijmer JG, Prins MH, Bonsel GJ, Bossuyt PM. The diagnostic odds ratio: a single indicator of test performance. J Clin Epidemiol. 2003;56:1129–35.
7. Habibzadeh F, Habibzadeh P, Yadollahie M. On determining the most appropriate test cut-off value: the case of tests with continuous results. Biochem Med (Zagreb). 2016;26:297–307.
8. Heston TF. Standardizing predictive values in diagnostic imaging research. J Magn Reson Imaging. 2011;33:505.

 9. Heston TF. Standardized predictive values. J Magn Reson Imaging. 2014;39:1338.
10. Hlatky MA, Mark DB, Harrell FE Jr, Lee KL, Califf RM, Pryor DB. Rethinking sensitivity and specificity. Am J Cardiol. 1987;59:1195–8.
11. Hsieh S, McGrory S, Leslie F, Dawson K, Ahmed S, Butler CR, et al. The Mini-Addenbrooke's Cognitive Examination: a new assessment tool for dementia. Dement Geriatr Cogn Disord. 2015;39:1–11.
12. Hunink MGM, Weinstein MC, Wittenberg E, Drummond MF, Pliskin JS, Wong JB, et al. Decision making in health and medicine. Integrating evidence and values. 2nd ed. Cambridge: Cambridge University Press; 2014.
13. Jaeschke R, Guyatt G, Sackett DL. Users' guide to the medical literature. III. How to use an article about a diagnostic test. B. What are the results and will they help me in caring for my patients? JAMA. 1994;271:703–7.
14. Kraemer HC. Evaluating medical tests. Objective and quantitative guidelines. Newbery Park: Sage; 1992.
15. Larner AJ. MACE for diagnosis of dementia and MCI: examining cut-offs and predictive values. Diagnostics (Basel). 2019;9:E51.
16. Larner AJ. Applying Kraemer's Q (positive sign rate): some implications for diagnostic test accuracy study results. Dement Geriatr Cogn Dis Extra. 2019;9:389–96.
17. Larner AJ. New unitary metrics for dementia test accuracy studies. Prog Neurol Psychiatry. 2019;23(3):21–5.
18. Larner AJ. Mini-Addenbrooke's Cognitive Examination (MACE): a useful cognitive screening instrument in older people? Can Geriatr J. 2020;23:199–204.
19. Larner AJ. The "attended alone" and "attended with" signs in the assessment of cognitive impairment: a revalidation. Postgrad Med. 2020;132:595–600.
20. Larner AJ. Cognitive screening instruments for dementia: comparing metrics of test limitation. medRxiv. 2020; https://doi.org/10.1101/2020.10.29.20222109v1.
21. Larner AJ. Manual of screeners for dementia. Pragmatic test accuracy studies. London: Springer; 2020.
22. Larrabee GJ, Barry DTR. Diagnostic classification statistics and diagnostic validity of malingering assessment. In: Larrabee GJ, editor. Assessment of malingered neuropsychological deficits. Oxford: Oxford University Press; 2007. p. 14–26.
23. Leeflang MM, Bossuyt PM, Irwig L. Diagnostic test accuracy may vary with prevalence: implications for evidence-based diagnosis. J Clin Epidemiol. 2009;62:5–12.
24. Leeflang MM, Rutjes AW, Reitsma JB, Hooft L, Bossuyt PM. Variation of a test's sensitivity and specificity with disease prevalence. CMAJ. 2013;185:E537–44.
25. Linn S. New patient-oriented diagnostic test characteristics analogous to the likelihood ratios conveyed information on trustworthiness. J Clin Epidemiol. 2005;58:450–7.
26. Mathuranath PS, Nestor PJ, Berrios GE, Rakowicz W, Hodges JR. A brief cognitive test battery to differentiate Alzheimer's disease and frontotemporal dementia. Neurology. 2000;55:1613–20.
27. McGee S. Simplifying likelihood ratios. J Gen Intern Med. 2002;17:647–50.
28. Mioshi E, Dawson K, Mitchell J, Arnold R, Hodges JR. The Addenbrooke's Cognitive Examination Revised: a brief cognitive test battery for dementia screening. Int J Geriatr Psychiatry. 2006;21:1078–85.
29. Mitchell AJ. Sensitivity x PPV is a recognized test called the clinical utility index (CUI+). Eur J Epidemiol. 2011;26:251–2.
30. Neyman J. Outline of statistical treatment of the problem of diagnosis. Public Health Rep. 1947;62:1449–56.
31. Ostergaard SD, Dinesen PT, Foldager L. Quantifying the value of markers in screening programmes. Eur J Epidemiol. 2010;25:151–4.
32. Perera R, Heneghan C. Making sense of diagnostic tests likelihood ratios. Evid Based Med. 2006;11:130–1.

33. Rosenthal JA. Qualitative descriptors of strength of association and effect size. J Soc Serv Res. 1996;21:37–59.
34. Schaefer JT. The critical success index as an indicator of warning skill. Weather Forecast. 1990;5:570–5.
35. Warrens MJ. A Kraemer-type rescaling that transforms the odds ratio into the weighted kappa coefficient. Psychometrika. 2010;75:328–30.
36. Yerushalmy J. Statistical problems in assessing methods of medical diagnosis, with special reference to x-ray techniques. Public Health Rep. 1947;62:1432–49.

# Chapter 3
# Paired Complementary Measures

## Contents

## 3.1   Introduction

This chapter considers complementary paired measures of discrimination. Conditional probability measures may be described as complementary (or negations) when they necessarily sum to unity. The summation principle that probabilities add to 1 holds for a mutually exclusive and exhaustive set of possibilities. This chapter reiterates some of the metrics previously examined in Chap. 2, as well as looking at other measures, namely accuracy and inaccuracy (Fig. 3.1). As in the previous chapter, the classification of measures as error-based and information-based, following Bossuyt [1], is used. Consideration is also given to correct classification and misclassification rates. The variation of paired measures with either the chosen cut-off or level of test (Q) or with the pre-test probability or prevalence (P) is also illustrated.

|  |  | True Status | | |
|---|---|---|---|---|
|  |  | **Condition present (= case)** | **Condition absent (= non case)** | $r^1$ |
| **Test Outcome** | **Positive** | True positive [TP] (a) | False positive [FP] (b) | q |
|  | **Negative** | **False negative [FN] (c)** | True negative [TN] (d) | $q^1$ |
|  |  | p | $p^1$ | r |

**Paired complementary measures (literal notation only):**

| | | | | |
|---|---|---|---|---|
| Sens (TPR) | = | TP/(TP + FN) | = | TP/p |
| FNR (1 – Sens) | = | FN/(TP + FN) | = | FN/p |
| Spec (TNR) | = | TN/(FP + TN) | = | TN/p' |
| FPR (1 – Spec) | = | FP/(FP + TN) | = | FP/p' |
| Acc | = | (TP + TN)/(TP + FP + FN + TN) | = | TP +TN/N |
| Inacc (1 – Acc) | = | FP + FN/(TP + FP + FN + TN) | = | FP + FN/N |
| PPV | = | TP/(TP + FP) | = | TP/q |
| FDR (1 – PPV) | = | FP/(TP + FP) | = | FP/q |
| NPV | = | TN/(FN + TN) | = | TN/q' |
| FRR (1 – NPV) | = | FN/(FN + TN) | = | FN/q' |

**Fig. 3.1**  $2 \times 2$ contingency table with literal and algebraic notation, marginal totals, and derived paired complementary measures

## 3.2  Error-Based Measures

### 3.2.1  *Sensitivity (Sens) and False Negative Rate (FNR)*

As previously mentioned (Sect. 2.2.3), false negative rate (FNR) is the complement of sensitivity (Sens):

$$FNR = (1 - Sens)$$
$$= (1 - TPR)$$

$$FNR + Sens = 1$$

$$FNR + TPR = 1$$

In error notation, FNR = $\beta$, Sens = $1 - \beta$.

This is illustrated in the worked examples of Sens (Sect. 2.2.1) and FNR (Sect. 2.2.3) from a study of the Mini-Addenbrooke's Cognitive Examination (MACE) [11] showing that the calculated values (Sens = 0.912, FNR = 0.088) sum to 1. Hence knowing either Sens or FNR will always disclose the other across the range of test cut-offs (i.e. variation with Q; Fig. 3.2).

**Fig. 3.2** Plot of Sensitivity (diamonds) and FNR (triangles) for dementia diagnosis at fixed P (= 0.151) on y axis versus MACE cut-off (x axis). (Data from [11])

This also holds for rescaled values [9, 12]:

$$\begin{aligned} FNR_Q &= (1-QSN) \\ &= (1-TPR_Q) \end{aligned}$$

In the same study of MACE (Sect. 2.2.2), QSN = 0.857 and so $FNR_Q$ = (1 − QSN) = 0.143.


## 3.2.2  Specificity (Spec) and False Positive Rate (FPR)

As previously mentioned (Sect. 2.2.3), false positive rate (FPR) is the complement of specificity (Spec):

$$\begin{aligned} FPR &= (1-Spec) \\ &= (1-TNR) \end{aligned}$$

$$\begin{aligned} FPR + Spec &= 1 \\ FPR + TNR &= 1 \end{aligned}$$

In error notation, FPR = $\alpha$, Spec = 1 − $\alpha$.

This is illustrated in the worked examples of Spec (Sect. 2.2.1) and FPR (Sect. 2.3.3) from the MACE study [11] showing that the calculated values (Spec = 0.707, FPR = 0.293) sum to 1. Hence knowing either Spec or FPR will always disclose the other across the range of test cut-offs (i.e. variation with Q; Fig. 3.3).

**Fig. 3.3** Plot of Specificity (diamonds) and FPR (triangles) for dementia diagnosis at fixed P (= 0.151) on y axis versus MACE cut-off (x axis). (Data from [11])

This also holds for rescaled values [9, 12]:

$$FPR_Q = (1-QSP)$$
$$= (1-TNR_Q)$$

In the same study of MACE (Sect. 2.2.2), QSP = 0.242 and so $FPR_Q = (1 - QSP)$ = 0.758.

### 3.2.3  "SnNout" and "SpPin" Rules

Gallagher [3] has suggested that the measures of sensitivity and specificity of diagnostic tests ask the wrong question from a clinician's point of view, since they presuppose that a patient either does or does not have a particular disease, in which case the administration of a diagnostic test would not be needed. The clinical utility of sensitivity and specificity is deemed to lie in the mathematical properties of these metrics [3].

A very sensitive test will have very few false negatives (but possibly many false positives). Because of the low FNR of a very sensitive test, a negative test result is therefore likely to be a true negative and hence rules out the diagnosis, as made explicit in the heuristic "SnNout" rule ([23], p.165–6):

Se̲nsitive test, N̲egative result, = diagnosis ruled ou̲t

Conversely, a test with low sensitivity has many false negatives, and hence misses cases.

A very specific test will have very few false positives (but possibly many false negatives). Because of the low FPR of a very specific test, a positive test result is therefore likely to be a true positive and hence rules in the diagnosis, as made explicit in the heuristic "SpPin" rule ([23], p.165–6):

$$\underline{Sp}ecific\ test, \underline{P}ositive\ result, \quad = \quad diagnosis\ ruled\ \underline{in}.$$

Conversely, a test with low specificity has many false positives, and hence mis-identifies non cases as cases.

### 3.2.4   Accuracy and Inaccuracy

Accuracy (Acc) is the sum of true positives and true negatives divided by the total number of patients tested. Acc ranges from 0 to 1, with higher values better.
In literal notation (Fig. 3.1):

$$
\begin{aligned}
Acc \quad &= \quad (TP+TN)/(TP+FP+FN+TN) \\
&= \quad (TP+TN)/N
\end{aligned}
$$

In algebraic notation:

$$
\begin{aligned}
Acc \quad &= \quad a+d/(a+b+c+d) \\
&= \quad a+d/N
\end{aligned}
$$

and in terms of marginal totals:

$$Acc \quad = \quad r/N$$

This is identical to the value R, defined as one of the marginal probabilities of the basic $2 \times 2$ contingency table (Sect. 1.3.2). Accuracy may also be known as correct classification accuracy, effectiveness rate, fraction correct (FC), test efficiency, or posterior probability, or may be stated as the number of individuals correctly classi-fied by the test. Accuracy, like diagnostic odds ratio (DOR; Sect. 2.4.1), treats FN and FP as equally undesirable, an assumption which is often not the case in clinical practice, and hence a shortcoming of this measure (see Sect. 3.2.5).

"Accuracy" is potentially an ambiguous term, as other measures of "accuracy" are also described [13], including the F measure (Sect. 4.9) and Matthews' correlation coefficient (Sect. 4.5), as well as the area under the receiver operating characteristic curve (Sect. 6.2).

Accuracy is calculated using values from both columns of the $2 \times 2$ contingency table and hence is sensitive to class imbalance or skews, or in other words it is dependent on disease prevalence, as a weighted average of sensitivity and specificity with weights related to sample prevalence (P and $1 - P$ or P'). Acc may therefore be expressed in terms of P, P', Sens and Spec, such that:

$$Acc \quad = \quad (Sens.P)+(Spec.P')$$

Hence in error notation:

$$Acc \quad = \quad (1-\beta).P + (1-\alpha).P'$$

Inaccuracy (Inacc), also sometimes known as error rate, or fraction incorrect, or misclassification rate (although this term has alternate usage; see Sect. 3.2.5), is the complement of Accuracy:

$$Inaccuracy \quad = \quad (1-Acc)$$

---

**Worked Example: Acc**
The Mini-Addenbrooke's Cognitive Examination (MACE) [7] was examined in a screening test accuracy study [11]. At the MACE cut-off of ≤20/30, TP = 104, FN =10, FP = 188, and TN = 453 (see Fig. 2.2).
  Hence the value for Acc at this cut-off is:

$$\begin{aligned} Acc \quad &= \quad (TP+TN)/(TP+FP+FN+TN) \\ &= \quad (104+453)/(104+188+10+453) \\ &= \quad 0.738 \end{aligned}$$

Acc may also be expressed in terms of P, P', Sens and Spec. In the MACE study [11], dementia prevalence (P) in the patient cohort (N = 755) was 0.151 (Sect. 1.3.2). Values for Sens and Spec at this MACE cut-off are 0.912 and 0.707 respectively (Sect. 2.2.1).
  Hence the value for Acc is:

$$\begin{aligned} Acc \quad &= \quad (Sens.P)+(Spec.P') \\ &= \quad (0.912\times0.151)+(0.707\times0.849) \\ &= \quad 0.738 \end{aligned}$$

---

Hence, Inacc ranges from 0 to 1 with lower values better. Inacc is given by the sum of false positives and false negatives divided by the total number of patients tested.

In literal notation (Fig. 3.1):

$$\begin{aligned} Inacc \quad &= \quad (FP+FN)/(TP+FP+FN+TN) \\ &= \quad (FP+FN)/N \end{aligned}$$

In algebraic notation:

$$\begin{aligned} Inacc \quad &= \quad b+c/(a+b+c+d) \\ &= \quad b+c/N \end{aligned}$$

and in terms of marginal totals:

$$\text{Inacc} \quad = \quad r'/N$$

This is identical to the value R′, defined as one of the marginal probabilities of the basic 2 × 2 contingency table (Sect. 1.3.2).

In terms of disease prevalence:

$$\text{Inacc} = (\text{FNR.P}) + (\text{FPR.P}')$$
$$= \left[(1 - \text{Sens}).P\right] + \left[(1 - \text{Spec}).P'\right]$$

Hence in error notation:

$$\text{Inacc} \quad = \quad (\beta.P) + (\alpha.P')$$

The reciprocal of inaccuracy has been defined as the "number needed to misdiagnose" (Sect. 5.4).

---

**Worked Example: Inacc**
In the screening test accuracy study of MACE [11], at the MACE cut-off of ≤20/30, TP = 104, FN =10, FP = 188, and TN = 453.
    Hence the value for Inacc at this cut-off is:

$$\text{Inacc} \quad = \quad (\text{FP} + \text{FN})/(\text{TP} + \text{FP} + \text{FN} + \text{TN})$$
$$= \quad (188 + 10)/(104 + 188 + 10 + 453)$$
$$= \quad 0.262$$

Inacc may also be expressed in terms of P, P′, FNR and FPR. Values for the latter two terms at this MACE cut-off are 0.088 and 0.293 respectively (Sect. 2.2.3).
    Hence the value for Inacc is:

$$\text{Inacc} \quad = \quad (\text{FNR.P}) + (\text{FPR.P}')$$
$$= \quad (0.088 \times 0.151) + (0.293 \times 0.849)$$
$$= \quad 0.262$$

---

Acc and Inacc are scalar values based on information from both columns of the 2 × 2 table (cf. Sens and Spec), hence vary with prevalence, P (Sect. 2.3.2), as well as with the level of the test, Q, and hence with test cut-off [11, 14] (Fig. 3.4), and are also sensitive to class imbalance.

As discussed previously (Sect. 2.2.1), Sens and Spec are unscaled measures, and hence so is Acc. As an unscaled measure, it gives no direct measure of the degree to which diagnostic uncertainty is reduced. This can be addressed by taking into

**Fig. 3.4** Plot of Accuracy (diamonds) and Inaccuracy (triangles) for dementia diagnosis at fixed P (= 0.151) on y axis versus MACE cut-off (x axis). (Data from [11])

account values of both P and Q, as for QSN and QSP (Sect. 2.2.2), to remove the biasing effects of random associations between test result and disease prevalence ([4], p.470), such that:

$$\text{Acc} = \left(\text{Sens.P} + \text{Spec.P}'\right) - \left(\text{P.Q} + \text{P}'.\text{Q}'\right)/1 - \left(\text{P.Q} + \text{P}'.\text{Q}'\right)$$

The latter, equivalent to the kappa statistic (Sect. 7.2.2), has a range 0 to 1, where 0 = ineffective test and 1 = perfect test.

**Worked Example: Unbiased Acc**

In the screening test accuracy study of MACE [11], dementia prevalence (P) was 0.151. The positive sign rate, Q = TP+FP/N, was 0.387 (Sect. 1.3.2).

At the MACE cut-off of ≤20/30, Sens = 0.912 and Spec = 0.707 (Sect. 2.2.1).

Hence the value for unbiased Acc at this MACE cut-off is:

$$
\begin{aligned}
\text{Acc} &= \left(\text{Sens.P} + \text{Spec.P}'\right) - \left(\text{P.Q} + \text{P}'.\text{Q}'\right)/1 - \left(\text{P.Q} + \text{P}'.\text{Q}'\right) \\
&= \left(0.138 + 0.600\right) - \left(0.058 + 0.520\right)/1 - \left(0.058 + 0.520\right) \\
&= 0.738 - 0.579/1 - 0.579 \\
&= 0.159/0.421 \\
&= 0.378
\end{aligned}
$$

Note how this differs from the standard calculation of Acc at this cut-off (= 0.738).

### 3.2.5   Classification and Misclassification Rates; Misclassification Costs

The consideration of the complementary paired measures of Sens and FNR (Sect. 3.2.1) and Spec and FPR (Sect. 3.2.2) prompts the inclusion here of a brief discussion of classification and misclassification.

Sens and Spec provide different pieces of information about a test. Is there some way to combine this information into a meaningful outcome parameter? One method has already been encountered, namely likelihood ratios (Sect. 2.3.4), and there are others including Youden index (Sect. 4.2) and receiver operating characteristic (ROC) curves (Sect. 6.2).

However, the simplest way to combine information about Sens and Spec is to sum them, a measure which has been termed "gain in certainty" [2] or overall correct classification rate [21].

$$\text{Correct classification rate} \;=\; \text{Sens} + \text{Spec}$$
$$=\; \text{TPR} + \text{TNR}$$

Of note, unlike most of the parameters considered so far, correct classification rate has a range of 0 to 2, with higher scores better (technically this is not, therefore, a "rate"). It has been argued that when Sens + Spec = 1 the test provides no information, whilst when the sum is greatest (i.e. = 2) the expected gain is maximised [2].

In literal notation (Fig. 3.1):

$$\text{Correct classification rate} \;=\; \left[\text{TP}/\left(\text{TP}+\text{FN}\right)\right]+\left[\text{TN}/\left(\text{FP}+\text{TN}\right)\right]$$
$$=\; \left[\text{TP}/\text{p}\right]+\left[\text{TN}/\text{p}'\right]$$

In algebraic notation:

$$\text{Correct classification rate} \;=\; \left[a/\left(a+c\right)\right]+\left[d/\left(b+d\right)\right]$$
$$=\; \left[a/\text{p}\right]+\left[d/\text{p}'\right]$$

In error notation (see Fig. 1.5):

$$\text{Correct classification rate} \;=\; \left(1-\beta\right)+\left(1-\alpha\right)$$

This summation of Sens and Spec is little used in clinical practice (e.g. [6], p.190; [17], p.100). The Youden index [24] is more frequently used (Sect. 4.2).

The term "misclassification rate" is potentially ambiguous, being sometimes used for the parameter called "proportion incorrect" (Sect. 1.3.2) or "inaccuracy" or "error rate" (Sect. 3.2.4). Here, the usage of Perkins and Schisterman [21] is followed:

$$\text{Misclassification rate} \;=\; \left(1-\text{Sens}\right)+\left(1-\text{Spec}\right)$$
$$=\; \text{FNR} + \text{FPR}$$
$$=\; 2-\left(\text{Sens}+\text{Spec}\right)$$

Misclassification rate has a range of 0 to 2, with lower scores better.
In literal notation (Fig. 3.1):

$$\text{Misclassification rate} = \left[FN/(FN+TP)\right]+\left[FP/(FP+TN)\right]$$
$$= \left[FN/p\right]+\left[FP/p'\right]$$

In algebraic notation:

$$\text{Misclassification rate} = \left[c/(a+c)\right]+\left[b/(b+d)\right]$$
$$= \left[c/p\right]+\left[b/p'\right]$$

In error notation (see Fig. 1.5):

$$\text{Misclassification rate} = \beta+\alpha$$

Hence correct classification rate and misclassification rate are negations which
sum to 2:

$$\text{Correct classification rate} + \text{Misclassification rate} = \text{Sens} + \text{Spec} + (1-\text{Sens})+(1-\text{Spec})$$
$$= 2$$

Their complement (sum to unity) is the Youden index (see Sect. 4.2).

Distinction should be drawn between this misclassification rate and another
parameter, called misclassification cost. Evidently, both FP and FN classifications
have costs (see also the discussion of net harm to net benefit (H/B) ratio in Sect.
2.3.5). In the context of diagnostic or screening test accuracy studies, it may be
argued that high test sensitivity in order to identify all true positives, hence with
very few false negatives, is more acceptable than tests with low sensitivity but high
specificity which risk false negatives (i.e. miss true positives), since the cost of a FN
error may be high. Indeed, Youden ([24], p.32) spoke of an "instinctive reaction
against a test that is subject to false negatives" since a missed diagnosis may mean
missed treatment with resulting disability and even death. This argument also
supposes that the cost of a FP error is not so serious: a healthy patient may be
subjected to extra screening and possibly inappropriate treatment unnecessarily.
However, the potential ramifications of FP error should not be underestimated, as
these may be "profoundly transformational on a personal level" ([18],
p.38–9,362,363).

Expected benefits (B) and costs (C) at each cut-off may be expressed as "expected
costs" (EC) [9, 22]:

$$EC = C_{FP} \times FP + C_{FN} \times FN - B_{TN} \times TN - B_{TP} \times TP$$

The test threshold, c*, with the lowest EC is optimal.

**Worked Example: Correct Classification Rate and Misclassification Rate**

In a screening test accuracy study of MACE [11], at the MACE cut-off of ≤20/30, values for Sens and Spec were 0.912 and 0.707 (Sect. 2.2.1) and hence for FPR and FNR were 0.293 and 0.088 respectively (Sect. 2.2.3).

Hence the value for the correct classification rate at this cut-off was:

$$
\begin{aligned}
\text{Correct classification rate} &= \text{TPR} + \text{TNR} \\
&= 0.912 + 0.707 \\
&= 1.619
\end{aligned}
$$

The value for the misclassification rate was:

$$
\begin{aligned}
\text{Misclassification rate} &= \text{FNR} + \text{FPR} \\
&= 0.088 + 0.293 \\
&= 0.381
\end{aligned}
$$

This may also be expressed as a cost ratio (Cr):

$$ Cr = B_{TP} - C_{FN} / B_{TP} + B_{TN} - C_{FN} - C_{FP} $$

The term $(B_{TP} - C_{FN})$ represents the difference in costs if patients with disease (D+) are classified correctly or not, whilst the term $(B_{TN} - C_{FP})$ represents the difference in costs if healthy individuals (D−) are classified correctly or not. Hence Cr is the costs for diseased relative to total costs, or the ratio of relative costs. Cr ranges from 0 to 1. When Cr = 0.5, the difference in costs between correct (T+) and incorrect (T−) test classification is equal for healthy (D−) and diseased (D+) persons. When Cr = 1, difference in costs is much higher for persons with disease (i.e. FN); when Cr = 0 the difference in costs is much higher for healthy persons (i.e. FP). In most disease screening situations, one anticipates Cr to tend toward 1, since FN errors have higher cost [22].

This notation may also be used in the expression of the net harm to net benefit (H/B) ratio (Sect. 2.3.5). As benefits may be expressed as negative costs if desired [19], and indeed all may be understood as cost expressions [8], then $B_{TP} = C_{TP}$ and $B_{TN} = C_{TN}$. Hence the term $C_{FP} - C_{TN}$ is equal to the net costs of treating a non-diseased patient (harm of FP), and the term $C_{FN} - C_{TP}$ is equal to the net benefits of treating a diseased patient [8] or net costs of not treating a diseased patient (harm of FN):

$$ \text{Net Harm} (H) / \text{Net Benefit} (B) = C_{FP} - C_{TN} / C_{FN} - C_{TP} $$

As the misclassification of non-diseased (FN) carries the highest cost, $C_{FN} \gg C_{TP}$, then ideally H/B ratio values should be as high as possible (Sect. 2.3.5).

The ratio of harms of FP to FN (treating a FP unnecessarily to not treating a TP) is also used in methods for determining optimal test cut-off from the receiver operating characteristic (ROC) curve (Sect. 6.2) [5].

Another term sometimes used is a relative misclassification cost, defined as FP/TP (literal notation) or b/a (algebraic notation). This is used, for example [20], in a method which gives weighting to the difference in Sens and Spec (ΔSens, ΔSpec) of two tests, hence a weighted comparison (WC), taking into account the relative misclassification cost of false positive diagnosis and also disease prevalence (P), as expressed in the equation:

$$WC = \Delta Sens + \left[ (1 - P / P) \times (FP / TP) \times \Delta Spec \right]$$

The relative misclassification cost, FP/TP, seeks to define how many false positives a true positive is worth, a potentially difficult estimate. An arbitrary value of FP/TP = 0.1 may be set [10, 16]. The WC equation does not ostensibly take false negatives into account, but the [(1 − P/P) x (FP/TP)] term resembles the net harm to net benefit (H/B) ratio definition (derived in Sect. 2.3.5), where the benefit of TP may be equated to the harm of a FN result.

The question of the relative cost of FP and FN also arises with respect to those metrics which assume FN and FP to be equally undesirable, e.g. DOR (Sect. 2.4.1), Acc (Sect. 3.2.4), and Youden index (Sect. 4.2). In all these situations, a trade-off between benefits and costs (sometimes painful) needs to be made.

## 3.3 Information-Based Measures

### 3.3.1 Positive Predictive Value (PPV) and False Discovery Rate (FDR)

As previously mentioned (Sect. 2.3.3), false discovery rate (FDR) is the complement of positive predictive value (PPV):

$$FDR \quad = \quad (1 - PPV)$$

This is illustrated in the worked examples of PPV (Sect. 2.3.1) and FDR (Sect. 2.3.3) from the MACE study [11] showing that the calculated values (PPV = 0.356, FDR = 0.644) sum to 1. Hence knowing either PPV or FDR will always disclose the other across the range of test cut-offs (i.e. variation with Q; Fig. 3.5).

This also holds for rescaled values [9, 12]:

$$FDR_Q \quad = \quad (1 - PPV_Q)$$

In the same study of MACE (Sect. 2.3.2), $PPV_Q = 0.356$ and so $FDR_Q = (1 - PPV_Q) = 0.644$.

**Fig. 3.5** Plot of PPV (diamonds) and FDR (triangles) for dementia diagnosis at fixed P (= 0.151) on y axis versus MACE cut-off (x axis). (Data from [11])

## 3.3.2   *Negative Predictive Value (NPV) and False Reassurance Rate (FRR)*

As previously mentioned (Sect. 2.3.3), false reassurance rate (FRR) is the complement of negative predictive value (NPV):

$$FRR \quad = \quad (1 - NPV)$$

This is illustrated in the worked examples of NPV (Sect. 2.3.1) and FRR (Sect. 2.3.3) from the MACE study [11] showing that the calculated values (NPV = 0.978, FRR = 0.022) sum to 1. Hence knowing either NPV or FRR will always disclose the other across the range of test cut-offs (i.e. variation with Q; Fig. 3.6).

This also holds for rescaled values [9, 12]:

$$FRR_Q \quad = \quad (1 - NPV_Q)$$

In the same study (Sect. 2.3.2), $NPV_Q = 0.978$ and so $FRR_Q = (1 - NPV_Q) = 0.022$.

Note from Fig. 3.6 that this is the only example in this chapter in which there is no cross-over between the complementary metrics, i.e. the ideal of separation is achieved. Clearly this is a consequence of the skewed nature of this particular dataset, with a very large number of true negatives and a very small number of false negatives.

**Fig. 3.6** Plot of NPV (diamonds) and FRR (triangles) for dementia diagnosis at fixed P (= 0.151) on y axis versus MACE cut-off (x axis). (Data from [11])

## 3.4    Dependence of Paired Complementary Measures on Prevalence (P)

Having illustrated the dependence of the various paired metrics on cut-off or Q at a fixed prevalence (Figs. 3.2, 3.3, 3.4, 3.5 and 3.6), here their dependence on prevalence (P) at a fixed Q is shown.

Whilst choosing the fixed value of P may be straightforward (the base rate of the study population), choosing a fixed value of Q may not be so evident. Options include maximal test accuracy, or maximal Youden index ([15], p.156–9 and 163–5). For the purposes of this illustration, maximal Youden index has been used (Sect. 4.2), which occurs at MACE cut-off ≤20/30.

Values for PPV and NPV may be calculated using Bayes' formula (Sect. 2.3.2):

$$
\begin{aligned}
\text{PPV} &= \text{Sens} \times P / (\text{Sens} \times P) + \left[ (1 - \text{Spec}) \times (1 - P) \right] \\
&= \text{Sens} \times P / (\text{Sens} \times P) + \left[ \text{FPR} \times (1 - P) \right]
\end{aligned}
$$

$$
\begin{aligned}
\text{NPV} &= \text{Spec} \times (1 - P) / \left[ \text{Spec} \times (1 - P) \right] + \left[ (1 - \text{Sens}) \times P \right] \\
&= \text{Spec} \times (1 - P) / \left[ \text{Spec} \times (1 - P) \right] + \left[ \text{FNR} \times P \right]
\end{aligned}
$$

FDR and FRR values are then the complements of PPV and NPV respectively. Values for Acc may be calculated using the equation (Sect. 3.2.4):

$$
\text{Acc} = (\text{Sens.P}) + (\text{Spec.P}')
$$

At MACE cut-off ≤20/30, this simplifies to:

$$\text{Acc} \;\; = \;\; 0.912.\text{P} + 0.707.\text{P}'$$

Inacc values are then the complements of Acc values.

Values for Sens and Spec at a fixed Q may be calculated using the equivalences (Sect. 2.3.2):

$$(\text{Sens} - \text{Q})/\text{Q}' = (\text{NPV} - \text{P}')/\text{P}$$

and

$$(\text{Spec} - \text{Q}')/\text{Q} = (\text{PPV} - \text{P})/\text{P}'$$

Hence:

$$\text{Sens} = \left[\text{Q}'.(\text{NPV} - \text{P}')/\text{P}\right] + \text{Q}$$

and

$$\text{Spec} = \left[\text{Q}.(\text{PPV} - \text{P})/\text{P}'\right] + \text{Q}'$$

FNR and FPR values are then the complements of Sens and Spec respectively.

Calculated values for Sens, FNR, Spec and FPR at 0.1 increments of P are shown in Table 3.1, and illustrated in Figs. 3.7 and 3.8. Similarly for values of Acc and Inacc in Table 3.2 and Fig. 3.9; and for PPV, FDR, NPV and FRR in Table 3.3 and Figs. 3.10 and 3.11.

These plots suggest that for this test accuracy study of MACE, test Spec, Acc and PPV are better at high prevalence whereas Sens and NPV are better at low prevalence. This pattern is the converse of that seen with Q, with Spec, Acc and PPV better at lower cut-offs (compare Figs. 3.3, 3.4 and 3.5 with Figs. 3.8, 3.9, and 3.10

**Table 3.1** Values of Sens, FNR, Spec, and FPR for dementia diagnosis at fixed MACE cut-off of ≤20/30 (= maximal Youden index; fixed Q = 0.387) at various prevalence levels

| P, P' | Sens | FNR | Spec | FPR |
|---|---|---|---|---|
| 0.1, 0.9 | 0.914 | 0.086 | 0.681 | 0.319 |
| 0.2, 0.8 | 0.908 | 0.092 | 0.728 | 0.272 |
| 0.3, 0.7 | 0.896 | 0.104 | 0.763 | 0.237 |
| 0.4, 0.6 | 0.884 | 0.116 | 0.790 | 0.210 |
| 0.5, 0.5 | 0.865 | 0.135 | 0.812 | 0.188 |
| 0.6, 0.4 | 0.840 | 0.160 | 0.830 | 0.170 |
| 0.7, 0.3 | 0.803 | 0.197 | 0.844 | 0.156 |
| 0.8, 0.2 | 0.746 | 0.254 | 0.857 | 0.143 |
| 0.9, 0.1 | 0.640 | 0.360 | 0.868 | 0.132 |

**Fig. 3.7** Plot of Sensitivity (diamonds) and FNR (triangles) for dementia diagnosis at fixed Q (= 0.387; MACE cut-off ≤20/30) on y axis versus prevalence P (x axis)

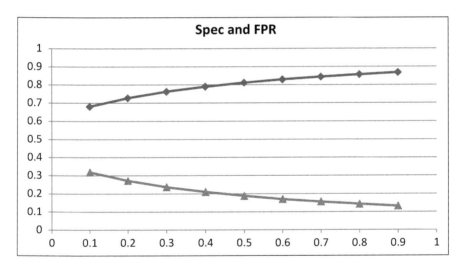

**Fig. 3.8** Plot of Specificity (diamonds) and FPR (triangles) for dementia diagnosis at fixed Q (= 0.387; MACE cut-off ≤20/30) on y axis versus prevalence P (x axis)

respectively) and Sens and NPV better at higher cut-offs (compare Figs. 3.2 and 3.6 with Figs. 3.7 and 3.11 respectively)

The interrelationship of P and Q may be illustrated by plotting a series of curves for different Q values against P. This is shown for Sens and Spec using the MACE dataset (Table 3.4, Figs. 3.12 and 3.13). At different selected MACE cut-offs (fixed

**Table 3.2** Values of Acc and Inacc for dementia diagnosis at fixed MACE cut-off of ≤20/30 (= maximal Youden index; fixed Q = 0.387) at various prevalence levels

| P, P′ | Acc | Inacc |
|---|---|---|
| 0.1, 0.9 | 0.728 | 0.272 |
| 0.2, 0.8 | 0.748 | 0.252 |
| 0.3, 0.7 | 0.769 | 0.231 |
| 0.4, 0.6 | 0.789 | 0.211 |
| 0.5, 0.5 | 0.810 | 0.190 |
| 0.6, 0.4 | 0.830 | 0.170 |
| 0.7, 0.3 | 0.851 | 0.149 |
| 0.8, 0.2 | 0.871 | 0.129 |
| 0.9, 0.1 | 0.892 | 0.108 |

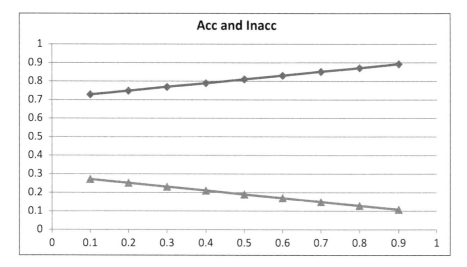

**Fig. 3.9** Plot of Accuracy (diamonds) and Inaccuracy (triangles) for dementia diagnosis at fixed Q (= 0.387; MACE cut-off ≤20/30) on y axis versus prevalence P (x axis)

**Table 3.3** Values of PPV, FDR, NPV, and FRR for dementia diagnosis at fixed MACE cut-off of ≤20/30 (= maximal Youden index; fixed Q = 0.387) at various prevalence levels

| P, P′ | PPV | FDR | NPV | FRR |
|---|---|---|---|---|
| 0.1, 0.9 | 0.257 | 0.743 | 0.986 | 0.014 |
| 0.2, 0.8 | 0.437 | 0.563 | 0.970 | 0.030 |
| 0.3, 0.7 | 0.571 | 0.429 | 0.949 | 0.051 |
| 0.4, 0.6 | 0.675 | 0.325 | 0.924 | 0.076 |
| 0.5, 0.5 | 0.757 | 0.243 | 0.890 | 0.110 |
| 0.6, 0.4 | 0.824 | 0.176 | 0.843 | 0.157 |
| 0.7, 0.3 | 0.879 | 0.121 | 0.775 | 0.225 |
| 0.8, 0.2 | 0.926 | 0.074 | 0.668 | 0.332 |
| 0.9, 0.1 | 0.966 | 0.034 | 0.472 | 0.528 |

**Fig. 3.10** Plot of PPV (diamonds) and FDR (triangles) for dementia diagnosis at fixed Q (= 0.387; MACE cut-off ≤20/30) on y axis versus prevalence P (x axis). Note equivalence of PPV curve to the conditional probability plot shown in Fig. 2.3.

**Fig. 3.11** Plot of NPV (diamonds) and FRR (triangles) for dementia diagnosis at fixed Q (= 0.387; MACE cut-off ≤20/30) on y axis versus prevalence P (x axis). Note equivalence of FRR curve to the conditional probability plot shown in Fig. 2.3.

values of Q and Q′) Sens and Spec were calculated (using the above equations) against variable P. Note that in this instance, PPV and NPV were also fixed for cut-off, and not recalculated for P (as in Table 3.1, Figs. 3.7 and 3.8). Again the finding is that, for this test accuracy study of MACE, Sens improves with increasing Q as P increases, and conversely Spec decreases with increasing Q as P increases. These

**Table 3.4**  Interrelationship of P and Q illustrated using data from MACE study [11]

| Cut-off | ≤14/30 | ≤17/30 | ≤20/30 | ≤23/30 | ≤26/30 |
|---|---|---|---|---|---|
| Q | 0.159 | 0.264 | 0.387 | 0.585 | 0.812 |
| Q′ | 0.841 | 0.736 | 0.613 | 0.415 | 0.188 |
| PPV | 0.558 | 0.422 | 0.356 | 0.253 | 0.184 |
| NPV | 0.926 | 0.946 | 0.978 | 0.994 | 0.993 |
| **Sens, Spec** | | | | | |
| **P, P′** | | | | | |
| 0.1, 0.9 | 0.378,0.922 | 0.603,0.830 | 0.865,0.723 | 0.975,0.514 | 0.986,0.264 |
| 0.2, 0.8 | 0.689,0.912 | 0.801,0.809 | 0.933,0.688 | 0.988,0.454 | 0.993,0.172 |
| 0.3, 0.7 | 0.793,0.900 | 0.868,0.782 | 0.955,0.644 | 0.992,0.376 | 0.996,0.053 |
| 0.4, 0.6 | 0.844,0.883 | 0.901,0.746 | 0.966,0.585 | 0.994,0.272 | 0.997, −0.104 |
| 0.5, 0.5 | 0.876,0.859 | 0.921,0.695 | 0.973,0.502 | 0.995,0.126 | 0.997, −0.325 |
| 0.6, 0.4 | 0.896,0.824 | 0.934,0.619 | 0.978,0.377 | 0.996, −0.09 | 0.998, −0.656 |
| 0.7, 0.3 | 0.911,0.766 | 0.943,0.491 | 0.981,0.169 | 0.996, −0.457 | 0.998, −1.21 |
| 0.8, 0.2 | 0.922,0.649 | 0.950,0.237 | 0.983, −0.246 | 0.997, −1.18 | 0.998, −2.31 |
| 0.9, 0.1 | 0.931,0.297 | 0.956, −0.526 | 0.985, −1.49 | 0.997, −3.37 | 0.999, −5.63 |

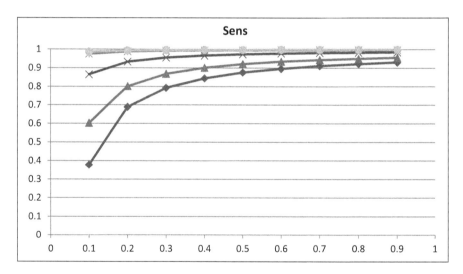

**Fig. 3.12**  Plot of Sens for five different MACE cut-offs (hence different values of Q) on y axis versus prevalence P (x axis); from data in Table 3.4

findings reflect the high sensitivity low specificity nature of MACE for dementia diagnosis [11]. Different findings may be anticipated with tests showing different performance characteristics (e.g. high sensitivity and high specificity, low sensitivity and high specificity).

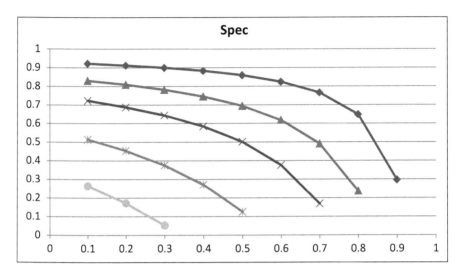

**Fig. 3.13** Plot of Spec for five different MACE cut-offs (hence different values of Q) on y axis versus prevalence P (x axis); from data in Table 3.4

# References

1. Bossuyt PMM. Clinical validity: defining biomarker performance. Scand J Clin Lab Invest. 2010;70(Suppl242):46–52.
2. Connell FA, Koepsell TD. Measures of gain in certainty from a diagnostic test. Am J Epidemiol. 1985;121:744–53.
3. Gallagher EJ. The problem with sensitivity and specificity.... Ann Emerg Med. 2003;42:298–303.
4. Garrett CT, Sell S. Summary and perspective: assessing test effectiveness – the identification of good tumour markers. In: Garrett CT, Sell S (eds.). Cellular cancer markers. Springer; 1995:455-477.
5. Habibzadeh F, Habibzadeh P, Yadollahie M. On determining the most appropriate test cut-off value: the case of tests with continuous results. Biochem Med (Zagreb). 2016;26:297–307.
6. Hancock P, Larner AJ. Clinical utility of Patient Health Questionnaire-9 (PHQ-9) in memory clinics. Int J Psychiatry Clin Pract. 2009;13:188–91.
7. Hsieh S, McGrory S, Leslie F, Dawson K, Ahmed S, Butler CR, et al. The Mini-Addenbrooke's Cognitive Examination: a new assessment tool for dementia. Dement Geriatr Cogn Disord. 2015;39:1–11.
8. Kaivanto K. Maximization of the sum of sensitivity and specificity as a diagnostic cutpoint criterion. J Cin Epidemiol. 2008;61:517–8.
9. Kraemer HC. Evaluating medical tests. Objective and quantitative guidelines. Newbery Park: Sage; 1992.
10. Larner AJ. Comparing diagnostic accuracy of cognitive screening instruments: a weighted comparison approach. Dement Geriatr Cogn Disord Extra. 2013;3:60–5.
11. Larner AJ. MACE for diagnosis of dementia and MCI: examining cut-offs and predictive values. Diagnostics (Basel). 2019;9:E51.
12. Larner AJ. Applying Kraemer's Q (positive sign rate): some implications for diagnostic test accuracy study results. Dement Geriatr Cogn Dis Extra. 2019;9:389–96.
13. Larner AJ. What is test accuracy? Comparing unitary accuracy metrics for cognitive screening instruments. Neurodegener Dis Manag. 2019;9:277–81.

14. Larner AJ. Defining "optimal" test cut-off using global test metrics: evidence from a cognitive screening instrument. Neurodegener Dis Manag. 2020;10:223–30.
15. Larner AJ. Manual of screeners for dementia. Pragmatic test accuracy studies. London: Springer; 2020.
16. Mallett S, Halligan S, Thompson M, Collins GS, Altman DG. Interpreting diagnostic accuracy studies for patient care. BMJ. 2012;345:e3999.
17. McCrea MA. Mild traumatic brain injury and postconcussion syndrome. The new evidence base for diagnosis and treatment. Oxford: Oxford University Press; 2008.
18. McKay RA. Patient Zero and the making of the AIDS epidemic. Chicago/London: University of Chicago Press; 2017.
19. Metz CE. Basic principles of ROC analysis. Semin Nucl Med. 1978;8:283–98.
20. Moons KGM, Stijnen T, Michel BC, Büller HR, Van Es GA, Grobbee DE, Habbema DF. Application of treatment thresholds to diagnostic-test evaluation: an alternative to the comparison of areas under receiver operating characteristic curves. Med Decis Making. 1997;17:447–54.
21. Perkins NJ, Schisterman EF. The inconsistency of "optimal" cutpoints obtained using two criteria based on the receiver operating characteristic curve. Am J Epidemiol. 2006;163:670–5.
22. Smits N. A note on Youden's J and its cost ratio. BMC Med Res Methodol. 2010;10:89.
23. Strauss SE, Glasziou P, Richardson WS, Haynes RB. Evidence-based medicine. How to practice and teach EBM. 5th ed. Edinburgh: Elsevier; 2019.
24. Youden WJ. Index for rating diagnostic tests. Cancer. 1950;3:32–5.

# Chapter 4
# Unitary Measures

## Contents

## 4.1 Introduction

In addition to the paired test metrics examined in chapters 2 and 3, there are also a number of global, single, or unitary metrics which may be used to summarise the outcomes of a 2 × 2 contingency table. Accuracy (Sect. 3.2.4) and diagnostic odds ratio (Sect. 2.4.1) are sometimes used as global outcome measures, but these are in fact paired (with inaccuracy and error odds ratio, respectively, although both the latter metrics are seldom used).

## 4.2 Youden Index (Y) or Statistic (J)

Youden [41] defined the Youden index (Y), or Youden J statistic, as:

$$Y = \text{Sens} + \text{Spec} - 1$$

Hence, like likelihood ratios (Sect. 2.3.4) and correct classification rate (Sect. 3.2.5), this is a metric which attempts to combine information from sensitivity (Sens) and specificity (Spec).

Values of Y may range from −1 to +1. However, most values of Y would be expected to fall within the range 0 (worthless, no diagnostic value) to 1 (perfect diagnostic value, no false positives or false negatives), with negative values

© Springer Nature Switzerland AG 2021
A. J. Larner, *The 2x2 Matrix*, https://doi.org/10.1007/978-3-030-74920-0_4

occurring only if the test were misleading, i.e. the test result was negatively associated with the true diagnosis. Y may be termed "informedness" in the informatics literature [34]. It has also been characterised as the maximum proportional reduction in expected "regret" achieved by a test, i.e. the difference in outcome between the action taken and the best action that could, in retrospect, have been taken [11].

Y may also be expressed in terms of false positive rate (FPR) and false negative rate (FNR) (Sect. 2.2.3) as:

$$
\begin{aligned}
Y &= \text{Sens} - (1 - \text{Spec}) \\
&= \text{Sens} - \text{FPR} \\
&= \text{TPR} - \text{FPR}
\end{aligned}
$$

or

$$
\begin{aligned}
Y &= \text{Spec} - (1 - \text{Sens}) \\
&= \text{Spec} - \text{FNR} \\
&= \text{TNR} - \text{FNR} \\
&= 1 - (\text{FPR} + \text{FNR})
\end{aligned}
$$

Hence Y is the difference between the two positive rates (TPR – FPR) or between the two negative rates (TNR – FNR). The outcomes of the addition of the two true rates (TPR + TNR) and of the two false rates (FNR + FPR), as the correct classification rate and the misclassification rate respectively, have previously been described (Sect. 3.2.5). Hence:

$$
\begin{aligned}
Y &= \text{Sens} + \text{Spec} - 1 \\
&= \text{TPR} + \text{TNR} - 1 \\
&= \text{Correct classification rate} - 1
\end{aligned}
$$

or

$$
\begin{aligned}
Y &= 1 \; (\text{FPR} + \text{FNR}) \\
&= 1 - \text{Misclassification rate}
\end{aligned}
$$

Y is therefore the complement or negation of the correct classification and misclassification rates (or the sum of the two false rates), with the end points of +1 and −1.

In literal notation (Fig. 1.1):

$$
\begin{aligned}
Y &= [\text{TP} / (\text{TP} + \text{FN})] + [\text{TN} / (\text{FP} + \text{TN})] - 1 \\
&= [\text{TP} / \text{p}] + [\text{TN} / \text{p}'] - 1
\end{aligned}
$$

Y may also be computed from the raw cell values from the $2 \times 2$ contingency table without first calculating Sens and Spec:

$$
Y = [(\text{TP} \times \text{TN}) - (\text{FP} \times \text{FN})] / [(\text{TP} + \text{FN})(\text{FP} + \text{TN})]
$$

In algebraic notation (Fig. 1.2):

$$Y = \left[a/(a+c)\right] + \left[d/(b+d)\right] - 1$$

or, without first calculating Sens and Spec:

$$Y = (ad - bc)/\left[(a+c).(b+d)\right]$$

or, in terms of marginal totals (Sect. 1.3.1):

$$Y = (ad - bc)/(p.p')$$

In error notation:

$$Y = (1-\beta) + (1-\alpha) - 1$$
$$= 1 - (\alpha + \beta)$$

Y can also be expressed in terms of likelihood ratios (Sect. 2.3.4):

$$
\begin{aligned}
Y &= \text{Sens} + \text{Spec} - 1 \\
&= (\text{LR}+ - 1) \times (1 - \text{Specificity}) \\
&= (\text{LR}+ - 1) \times \text{FPR} \\
&= (1 - \text{LR}-) \times \text{Specificity} \\
&= (\text{LR}+ - 1) \times (1 - \text{LR}-)/(\text{LR}+ - \text{LR}-)
\end{aligned}
$$

For the particular case of a single-threshold binary classifier, there is also a method to calculate Y from the area under the receiver operating characteristic (ROC) plot (see Sect. 6.2).

Y varies with test cut-off (Fig. 4.1) [16, 20].

---

**Worked Examples: Youden Index (Y)**

The Mini-Addenbrooke's Cognitive Examination (MACE) [12] was subjected to a screening test accuracy study [16]. At the MACE cut-off of ≤20/30, TP = 104, FN =10, FP = 188, and TN = 453 (Fig. 2.2).

Hence the values for Sens and Spec are (Sect. 2.2.1):

$$
\begin{aligned}
\text{Sens} &= \text{TP}/(\text{TP}+\text{FN}) \\
&= 104/(104+10) \\
&= 0.912
\end{aligned}
$$

$$
\begin{aligned}
\text{Spec} &= \text{TN}/(\text{TN}+\text{FP}) \\
&= 453/(453+188) \\
&= 0.707
\end{aligned}
$$

Therefore the value for Y is:

$$Y = \text{Sens} + \text{Spec} - 1$$
$$= 0.912 + 0.707 - 1$$
$$= 0.619$$

Examining all test cut-offs, this was the cut-off giving the maximal value for Youden index for dementia diagnosis [16] (hence use of this cut-off in previous worked examples).

Y may also be calculated without first knowing Sens and Spec:

$$Y = \left[(TP \times TN) - (FP \times FN)\right] / \left[(TP + FN)(FP + TN)\right]$$
$$= \left[(104 \times 453) - (188 \times 10)\right] / \left[(104 + 10)(188 + 453)\right]$$
$$= 45232 / 73074$$
$$= 0.619$$

It was previously shown (Sect. 2.3.4) that LR+ = 3.11 and LR- = 0.124 at MACE cut-off $\leq 20/30$. Expressing Y in terms of LRs:

$$Y = (LR+ - 1) \times (1 - LR-) / (LR+ - LR-)$$
$$= (3.11 - 1) \times (1 - 0.124) / (3.11 - 0.124)$$
$$= 2.11 \times 0.876 / 2.986$$
$$= 0.619$$

It was also previously shown (Sect. 3.2.5) that Correct classification rate was 1.619, hence Y = Correct classification rate – 1

It was also shown (Sect. 3.2.5) that Misclassification rate was 0.381, hence Y = 1 – Misclassification rate.

Y has some shortcomings as a global measure [17]. Being derived from Sens and Spec, strict columnar ratios, it would be anticipated that Y, like Sens and Spec, is independent of prevalence. Certainly Youden ([41], p.33) stated that Y was independent of the size, relative or absolute, of the control and disease groups. In practice, Sens and Spec, and hence Y, are not independent of disease prevalence [2], as is shown for the MACE study in Table 4.1 and Fig. 4.2 which indicate that in this dataset Y is optimal at $P = 0.5$. Moreover, Y implicitly employs a ratio of misclassification costs for FN and FP which varies with prevalence and so Y is not truly optimal [39]. Its maximal value arbitrarily assumes disease prevalence to be 50%, and treats FN and FP as equally undesirable, which is often not the case in clinical practice. In terms of cost ratio (Sect. 3.2.5), Y assumes $Cr = 0.5$, i.e. that the

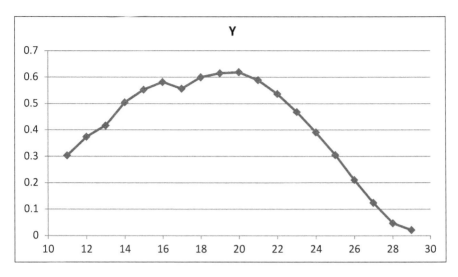

**Fig. 4.1**  Plot of Youden index (y axis) for dementia diagnosis at fixed P (= 0.151) versus MACE cut-off (x axis) [19]

**Table 4.1**  Values of Sens, Spec (from Table 3.1), and Y for dementia diagnosis at fixed MACE cut-off of ≤20/30 at various prevalence levels

| P, P′ | Sens | Spec | Y |
|---|---|---|---|
| 0.1, 0.9 | 0.914 | 0.681 | 0.595 |
| 0.2, 0.8 | 0.908 | 0.728 | 0.636 |
| 0.3, 0.7 | 0.896 | 0.763 | 0.659 |
| 0.4, 0.6 | 0.884 | 0.790 | 0.674 |
| 0.5, 0.5 | 0.865 | 0.812 | 0.677 |
| 0.6, 0.4 | 0.840 | 0.830 | 0.670 |
| 0.7, 0.3 | 0.803 | 0.844 | 0.647 |
| 0.8, 0.2 | 0.746 | 0.857 | 0.603 |
| 0.9, 0.1 | 0.640 | 0.868 | 0.508 |

difference in costs between correct and incorrect test classification is equal for both the healthy and diseased [39].

Y has an application in defining optimal test cut-off from the receiver operating characteristic (ROC) curve (Sect. 6.2.1) [38].

Y may be rescaled according to the level of the test, Q (see Sect. 2.2.2), such that [18]:

$$Y_Q = QSN + QSP - 1$$

The reciprocal (multiplicative inverse) of Y has been termed the number needed to diagnose (NND) [27] (see Sect. 5.2).

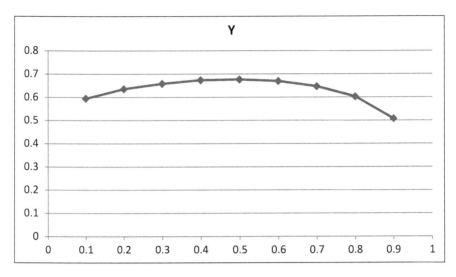

**Fig. 4.2** Plot of Youden index (y axis) for dementia diagnosis at fixed Q (MACE cut-off ≤20/30) versus prevalence P (x axis)

## 4.3    Predictive Summary Index (PSI, Ψ)

Linn and Grunau [27] defined the predictive summary index (PSI, Ψ), combining positive and negative predictive values (Sect. 2.3.1), as:

$$PSI \ = \ PPV + NPV - 1$$

Values of PSI may range from −1 to +1. However, most values of PSI would be expected to fall within the range 0 (no diagnostic value) to 1 (perfect predictive value, no false discoveries or false reassurances), with negative values occurring only if the test were misleading, i.e. the test result was negatively associated with the true diagnosis. PSI may be termed "markedness" in the informatics literature [34].

PSI may also be expressed in terms of false discovery rate (FDR) and false reassurance rate (FRR) (Sect. 2.3.3) as:

$$
\begin{aligned}
PSI &= \ PPV - (1 - NPV) \\
&= \ PPV - FRR \\
&= \ NPV - (1 - PPV) \\
&= \ NPV - FDR
\end{aligned}
$$

This measure may be characterised as the net gain of certainty of a test, by summing gain in certainty that a condition is either present or absent:

$$
\begin{aligned}
PSI &= \ (PPV - P) + \left[ NPV - (1 - P) \right] \\
&= \ PPV + NPV - 1
\end{aligned}
$$

In literal notation (Fig. 1.1):

$$\begin{aligned} PSI &= \left[TP/(TP+FP)\right]+\left[TN/(FN+TN)\right]-1 \\ &= \left[TP/q\right]+\left[TN/q'\right]-1 \end{aligned}$$

In algebraic notation (Fig. 1.2):

$$PSI = \left[a/(a+b)\right]+\left[d/(c+d)\right]-1$$

PSI may also be computed from the raw cell values from the 2 × 2 contingency table without first calculating PPV and NPV:

$$PSI = \left[(TP\times TN)-(FP\times FN)\right]/\left[(TP+FP)(FN+TN)\right]$$

In algebraic notation:

$$PSI = (ad-bc)/\left[(a+b).(c+d)\right]$$

and in terms of marginal totals:

$$PSI = (ad-bc)/(q.q')$$

**Worked Examples: Predictive Summary Index (PSI or Ψ)**
In a screening test accuracy study of MACE [16], at the MACE cut-off giving maximal Youden index for dementia diagnosis, ≤20/30, TP = 104, FN =10, FP = 188, and TN = 453.
Hence the values for PPV and NPV at this cut-off are (Sect. 2.3.1):

$$\begin{aligned} PPV &= TP/(TP+FP) \\ &= 104/(104+188) \\ &= 0.356 \end{aligned}$$

$$\begin{aligned} NPV &= TN/(TN+FN) \\ &= 453/(453+10) \\ &= 0.978 \end{aligned}$$

Therefore the value for PSI is:

$$\begin{aligned} PSI &= PPV+NPV-1 \\ &= 0.356+0.978-1 \\ &= 0.334 \end{aligned}$$

PSI may also be calculated without first knowing PPV and NP:

$$\begin{aligned} PSI &= \left[(TP \times TN) - (FP \times FN)\right] / \left[(TP + FP)(FN + TN)\right] \\ &= \left[(104 \times 453) - (188 \times 10)\right] / \left[(104 + 188)(10 + 453)\right] \\ &= 45232 / 135196 \\ &= 0.334 \end{aligned}$$

PSI varies with test cut-off or Q (Fig. 4.3) [16], with a different maximal cut-off value from Y.

PSI also varies with prevalence, as shown for the MACE study in Table 4.2 and Fig. 4.4, with optimal PSI at P = 0.6 (cf. Y, optimal at P = 0.5).

It has been argued that PSI may be useful for making population-based policy decisions, but that it adds little useful information to practicing clinicians attempting to apply research findings to individual patients [10].

The reciprocal (multiplicative inverse) of PSI has been termed the number needed to predict (NNP) [27] (see Sect. 5.3).

## 4.4   Harmonic Mean of Y and PSI (HMYPSI)

Just as Youden's index (Y) is an attempt to combine information about Sens and Spec, as are likelihood ratios (Sect. 2.3.4) and the receiver operating characteristic (ROC) curve (Sect. 6.2), and as predictive summary index (PSI) is an attempt to

**Fig. 4.3**  Plot of PSI (y axis) for dementia diagnosis at fixed P (= 0.151) versus MACE cut-off (x axis) (data from [15])

**Table 4.2**  Values of PPV, NPV (from Table 3.3), and PSI for dementia diagnosis at fixed MACE cut-off of ≤20/30 at various prevalence levels

| P, P′ | PPV | NPV | PSI |
|---|---|---|---|
| 0.1, 0.9 | 0.257 | 0.986 | 0.243 |
| 0.2, 0.8 | 0.437 | 0.970 | 0.407 |
| 0.3, 0.7 | 0.571 | 0.949 | 0.520 |
| 0.4, 0.6 | 0.675 | 0.924 | 0.599 |
| 0.5, 0.5 | 0.757 | 0.890 | 0.647 |
| 0.6, 0.4 | 0.824 | 0.843 | 0.667 |
| 0.7, 0.3 | 0.879 | 0.775 | 0.654 |
| 0.8, 0.2 | 0.926 | 0.668 | 0.594 |
| 0.9, 0.1 | 0.966 | 0.472 | 0.438 |

**Fig. 4.4**  Plot of PSI (y axis) for dementia diagnosis at fixed Q (MACE cut-off ≤20/30) on versus prevalence P (x axis)

combine information about predictive values, it may also be helpful to have measures which attempt to combine Sens and Spec and predictive values. Options include the clinical utility indexes (Sect. 2.4.2) and the summary utility index (Sect. 4.10).

Another option is the mean of Y and PSI, either geometric, which is the Matthews' correlation coefficient (MCC; Sect. 4.5), or harmonic, since geometric and harmonic means have advantages over the arithmetic mean in skewed datasets. To my knowledge, the latter has attracted no particular name, so I use the term "harmonic mean of Y and PSI" or HMYPSI, where:

$$\text{HMYPSI} = 2/\left[1/Y + 1/\text{PSI}\right]$$
$$= 2.\text{Y}.\text{PSI}/\left(Y + \text{PSI}\right)$$

**Worked Example: Harmonic Mean of Y and PSI (HMYPSI)**
In the screening test accuracy study of MACE [16], at the MACE cut-off of
$\leq 20/30$ the value of Y = 0.619 (Sect. 4.2) and of PSI = 0.334 (Sect. 4.3).

$$
\begin{aligned}
\text{HMYPSI} \;&=\; 2.\text{Y}.\text{PSI}/(\text{Y}+\text{PSI}) \\
&=\; 2\times 0.619\times 0.334 / (0.619+0.334) \\
&=\; 0.413/0.953 \\
&=\; 0.433
\end{aligned}
$$

Like Y and PSI, the value of HMYPSI may range from $-1$ to $+1$, with higher
values better.

HMYPSI values vary with test cut-off or Q (Fig. 4.5), with maximal cut-off
closer to that of PSI than to that of Y.

HMYPSI values also vary with prevalence (Table 4.3, Fig. 4.6).

In one particular case, when b = c in the 2 × 2 contingency table (Fig. 1.2; i.e.
false positives = false negatives), and hence the marginal totals align (i.e. the matrix
is symmetric), such that (a + b) = (a + c) and (b + d) = (c + d), then the values of
HMYPSI and MCC coincide (in terms of marginal totals, when p = q and p' = q').
In this situation, HMYPSI would also coincide with the value of the kappa statistic
(Sect. 7.2.2).

**Fig. 4.5** Plot of HMYPSI (y axis) for dementia diagnosis at fixed P (= 0.151) versus MACE cut-off (x axis)

**Table 4.3**  Values of Y (from Table 4.1), PSI (from Table 4.2), HMYPSI and MCC for dementia diagnosis at fixed MACE cut-off of ≤20/30 at various prevalence levels

| P, P′ | Y | PSI | HMYPSI | MCC |
|---|---|---|---|---|
| 0.1, 0.9 | 0.595 | 0.243 | 0.345 | 0.380 |
| 0.2, 0.8 | 0.636 | 0.407 | 0.496 | 0.509 |
| 0.3, 0.7 | 0.659 | 0.520 | 0.581 | 0.585 |
| 0.4, 0.6 | 0.674 | 0.599 | 0.634 | 0.635 |
| 0.5, 0.5 | 0.677 | 0.647 | 0.662 | 0.662 |
| 0.6, 0.4 | 0.670 | 0.667 | 0.668 | 0.668 |
| 0.7, 0.3 | 0.647 | 0.654 | 0.650 | 0.650 |
| 0.8, 0.2 | 0.603 | 0.594 | 0.598 | 0.598 |
| 0.9, 0.1 | 0.508 | 0.438 | 0.470 | 0.472 |

**Fig. 4.6**  Plot of HMYPSI (y axis) for dementia diagnosis at fixed Q (MACE cut-off ≤20/30) versus prevalence P (x axis)

## 4.5   Matthews' Correlation Coefficient (MCC)

Matthews [28] defined a correlation coefficient (MCC).
   In literal notation:

$$MCC = \left[(TP \times TN) - (FP \times FN)\right] / \sqrt{\left[(TP + FP)(TP + FN)(TN + FP)(TN + FN)\right]}$$

   In algebraic notation:

$$MCC = \left[(a \times d) - (b \times c)\right] / \sqrt{\left[(a+b).(a+c).(b+d).(c+d)\right]}$$
$$= (ad - bc) / \sqrt{(q.p.p'.q')}$$

MCC is equivalent to the Pearson phi ($\varphi$) coefficient, an effect size from the family of measures of association (Sect. 6.4)

MCC is also the geometric mean of the Youden index (Y) or informedness (Sect. 4.2) and the predictive summary index (PSI) or markedness (Sect. 4.3):

$$MCC = \sqrt{(Y \times PSI)}$$

For those geometrically minded, calculation of MCC may be related to a theorem in elementary geometry: for a right triangle, ABC, the perpendicular AD divides BC into two portions, BD and DC. The length of the perpendicular AD = $\sqrt{(BD \times DC)}$, the geometric mean of BD and DC. If we substitute Y and PSI for BD and DC, then AD = MCC.

The geometric mean is preferred to the arithmetic mean in skewed datasets, as is the harmonic mean (Sect. 4.4).

MCC has a range of $-1$ to $+1$, where $+1$ represents perfect prediction, 0 is no better than random, and $-1$ indicates total disagreement between prediction and observation.

For ease of comparison with other accuracy metrics, a normalised MMC (nMMC), with range 0 to 1, may be calculated [4], as:

$$nMCC = (MMC+1)/2$$

**Worked Examples: Matthews' Correlation Coefficient (MCC)**
In a screening test accuracy study of the MACE in a cohort of 755 consecutive patients [16], at the cut-off for dementia diagnosis of $\leq 20/30$, TP = 104, FN =10, FP = 188, and TN = 453.
Hence the value for MCC is:

$$MCC = [(TP \times TN) - (FP \times FN)] / \sqrt{\begin{bmatrix} (TP+FP)(TP+FN) \\ (TN+FP)(TN+FN) \end{bmatrix}}$$

$$= [(104 \times 453) - (188 \times 10)] / \sqrt{\begin{bmatrix} (104+188)(104+10) \\ (188+453)(10+453) \end{bmatrix}}$$

$$= 45232 / 99394.73$$

$$= 0.455$$

It was previously shown for MACE at this cut-off that Y = 0.619 (Sect. 4.2) and PSI = 0.334 (Sect. 4.3).
Hence the value for MCC may also be calculated as:

$$MCC = \sqrt{(Y \times PSI)}$$

$$= \sqrt{(0.619 \times 0.334)}$$

$$= 0.455$$

The value for nMCC is:

$$nMCC = (MCC + 1) / 2$$
$$= (0.455 + 1) / 2$$
$$= 0.727$$

MCC values vary with test cut-off [20] in a pattern almost identical to that shown for HMYPSI (Fig. 4.5), with the same maximal cut-off (Table 6.2). Likewise, the variation of MCC with prevalence is almost identical to that for HMYPSI (Table 4.3), diverging only at the extremes.

MCC values have been calculated for several cognitive screening instruments and appear to be the least optimistic compared to Acc, area under the receiver operating characteristic curve (AUC ROC), and the F measure [19].

MCC is widely regarded as being a very informative score for establishing the quality of a binary classifier, since it takes into account the size of all four classes in the table, and allows for imbalanced data [1, 3, 4]. Hence it may be preferred to F measure (Sect. 4.9) [4].

## 4.6   Identification Index (II)

Mitchell [29] proposed an identification index (II) based on Accuracy and Inaccuracy (Sect. 3.2.4):

$$
\begin{aligned}
II &= \text{Acc} - \text{Inacc} \\
&= \text{Acc} - (1 - \text{Acc}) \\
&= 2.\text{Acc} - 1
\end{aligned}
$$

As Acc ranges from 0 to 1, and is the complement or negation of Inacc, II has a range of $-1$ to $+1$, with most scores anticipated in the range 0 to $+1$.

In literal notation:

$$
\begin{aligned}
II &= 2\left[ (TP + TN) / (TP + FP + FN + TN) \right] - 1 \\
&= 2\left[ (TP + TN) / N \right] - 1
\end{aligned}
$$

In algebraic notation:

$$
\begin{aligned}
II &= 2(a + d) / (a + b + c + d) - 1 \\
&= 2\left[ (a + d) / N \right] - 1
\end{aligned}
$$

**Worked Example: Identification Index (II)**
In a screening test accuracy study of MACE [16], at the MACE cut-off giving maximal Youden index for dementia diagnosis, $\leq 20/30$, TP = 104, FN =10, FP = 188, and TN = 453.

Hence the value for Acc (Sect. 3.2.4) at this cut-off is:

$$
\begin{aligned}
\text{Acc} &= (\text{TP} + \text{TN}) / (\text{TP} + \text{FN} + \text{FP} + \text{TN}) \\
&= (104 + 453) / (104 + 10 + 188 + 453) \\
&= 0.738
\end{aligned}
$$

Therefore the value for II is:

$$
\begin{aligned}
\text{II} &= 2.\text{Acc} - 1 \\
&= (2 \times 0.738) - 1 \\
&= 0.475
\end{aligned}
$$

In terms of marginal totals:

$$
\text{II} = 2(r/N) - 1
$$

Acc and, hence, II both vary with the chosen test cut-off [16].

The reciprocal (multiplicative inverse) of II has been termed the number needed to screen (NNS) [29] (Sect. 5.6).

## 4.7   Net Reclassification Improvement (NRI)

Net reclassification improvement or net reclassification index (NRI) may be used to quantify test performance. NRI expresses the change in the proportion of correct classification based on an investigation that has been added to the existing diagnostic information [32]. Most simply, this may be calculated as the difference between prior (pre-test) probability of diagnosis, or prevalence, P (Sect. 1.3.2), and posterior probability or test accuracy, Acc (Sect. 3.2.4) [36]:

$$
\begin{aligned}
\text{NRI} &= \text{posterior probability} - \text{pre-test probability} \\
&= \text{Accuracy} - \text{Prevalence} \\
&= \text{Acc} - \text{P}
\end{aligned}
$$

NRI is claimed to be intuitive and easy to use [36]. Evidently, a highly accurate test may be associated with small NRI if P is high, and a low accuracy test may be associated with large NRI if P is low.

In literal notation (Fig. 1.1):

$$
\begin{aligned}
NRI &= \left[(TP+TN)/(TP+FP+FN+TN)\right]-\left[(TP+FN)/N\right] \\
&= \left[(TP+TN)/N\right]-\left[(TP+FN)/N\right] \\
&= (TN-FN)/N
\end{aligned}
$$

In algebraic notation (Fig. 1.2):

$$
\begin{aligned}
NRI &= \left[(a+d)/(a+b+c+d)\right]-(a+c)/N \\
&= \left[(a+d)/N\right]-\left[(a+c)/N\right] \\
&= (d-c)/N
\end{aligned}
$$

In terms of marginal totals:

$$
\begin{aligned}
NRI &= r/N-p/N \\
&= R-P
\end{aligned}
$$

---

**Worked Example: Net Reclassification Improvement (NRI)**
In a screening test accuracy study of MACE [16], in a cohort of 755 consecutive patients the prevalence of dementia was $114/755 = 0.151$ (Sect. 1.3.2). At the MACE cut-off giving maximal Youden index for dementia diagnosis, $\leq 20/30$, TP = 104, FN =10, FP = 188, and TN = 453, Acc was 0.738 (Sect. 3.2.4).
   Hence the value for NRI at this cut-off is:

$$
\begin{aligned}
NRI &= Acc-P \\
&= 0.738-0.151 \\
&= 0.587
\end{aligned}
$$

or

$$
\begin{aligned}
NRI &= (TN-FN)/N \\
&= (453-10)/755 \\
&= 0.587
\end{aligned}
$$

---

Other usages of "net reclassification improvement" based on reclassification tables may be used ([13], p.199–201).

## 4.8    Critical Success Index (CSI) or Threat Score (TS)

The critical success index (CSI) [37], or threat score (TS) [31], or ratio of verification [9], is sometimes used in the context of weather forecasting, and has been defined as the ratio of hits to the sum of hits, false alarms, and misses. This might also be characterised (Sect. 1.2) as the ratio of true positives to the sum of true positives, false positives, and false negatives.

In literal notation:

$$CSI = TP/(TP+FN+FP)$$

In algebraic notation:

$$CSI = a/(a+b+c)$$

CSI may also be expressed in terms of Sens and PPV:

$$CSI = 1/[(1/PPV)+(1/Sens)-1]$$

CSI ranges from 0 to 1 (perfect forecast).

**Worked Examples: Critical Success Index (CSI)**
In a screening test accuracy study of MACE [16], the MACE cut-off giving maximal Youden index for dementia diagnosis was $\leq20/30$, where TP = 104, FN = 10, and FP = 188.

Hence the value for CSI is:

$$\begin{aligned} CSI &= TP/(TP+FN+FP) \\ &= 104/(104+10+188) \\ &= 0.344 \end{aligned}$$

In the screening test accuracy study of MACE, the values for Sens and PPV at cut-off $\leq20/30$ were 0.912 (Sect. 2.2.1) and 0.356 (Sect. 2.3.1) respectively.

Hence the value for CSI calculated using these measures is:

$$\begin{aligned} CSI &= 1/[(1/PPV)+(1/Sens)-1] \\ &= 1/[(1/0.356)+(1/0.912)-1] \\ &= 1/2.905 \\ &= 0.344 \end{aligned}$$

Ignoring TN (= 453), the calculated CSI suggests MACE is a poor forecaster of the diagnosis of dementia at this cut-off.

Obviously CSI ignores true negatives (TN, or d), or correct "non-events". Part of the rationale for the initial development of the critical success index was to avoid over-inflation of test metrics as a consequence of very large numbers of true negatives [9] (i.e. class skew or imbalance), for example metrics such as specificity (= d/(b+d)) and correct classification accuracy (= (a+d)/N).

CSI is not unbiased, since CSI = TP/(N − TN) = a/(N − d), and hence gives lower scores for rarer events. To offset this, a related score may be used to account for hits expected by chance. This is the equitable threat score (ETS) [8], also known as the Gilbert skill score [37]:

$$ETS = a - a_r / (a + b + c - a_r)$$

where

$$a_r = (\text{total forecasts of event}).(\text{total observations of event})/\text{sample size}$$

In literal notation:

$$a_r = (TP + FP)(TP + FN)/N$$

In algebraic notation:

$$a_r = (a + b).(a + c)/N$$

In terms of marginal totals:

$$a_r = q.p/N$$

Substituting, in literal notation:

$$ETS = \left[ TP - (TP + FP).(TP + FN)/N \right] / \left[ TP + FN + FP - (TP + FP).(TP + FN)/N \right]$$

In algebraic notation:

$$ETS = \left[ a - (a + b).(a + c)/N \right] / \left[ a + b + c - (a + b).(a + c)/N \right]$$

In terms of marginal totals:

$$ETS = (a - q.p/N)/(a + b + c - q.p/N)$$

This correction for chance is analogous to that used in the kappa statistic (Sect. 7.2.2). ETS values range from $-1/3$ to 1, and are lower than CSI values.

**Worked Example: Equitable Threat Score (ETS)**
In a screening test accuracy study of MACE [16], the MACE cut-off giving
maximal Youden index for dementia diagnosis was ≤20/30, where TP = 104,
FN =10, and FP = 188.
Hence the value for $a_r$ is:

$$
\begin{aligned}
a_r &= (TP + FP).(TP + FN)/N \\
    &= (104 + 188).(104 + 10)/755 \\
    &= 44.09
\end{aligned}
$$

Substituting, the value for ETS is:

$$
\begin{aligned}
ETS &= TP - a_r /(TP + FN + FP) - a_r \\
    &= (104 - 44.09)/(104 + 10 + 188) - 44.09 \\
    &= 0.232
\end{aligned}
$$

The calculated ETS suggests MACE is a poor forecaster of diagnosis of
dementia at this cut-off, as for CSI.

To my knowledge, CSI and ETS values have only recently been used in the char-
acterisation of cognitive screening test accuracy studies [26], but as the examples
show they are easy to calculate. Both values vary with test cut-off or Q (Fig. 4.7),
with maximum identical to HMYPSI and MCC in this dataset (Table 6.2).

**Fig. 4.7** Plot of CSI (diamonds) and ETS (triangles) on y-axis versus MACE cut-off (x axis) [25]

## 4.9   F Measure (F) or F1 Score (Dice Coefficient)

The F measure (F) or F1 score [34, 35] is defined as the harmonic mean of precision or positive predictive value (PPV; Sect. 2.3.1) and sensitivity or recall (Sect. 2.2.1). This corresponds to the coefficient described by Dice in 1948 [7], and independently by Sørensen [40], itself a reinvention of a metric described by Jaccard in 1901 (in French; translated into English in 1912 [14]).

$$F = 2.PPV.Sens / (PPV + Sens)$$
$$= 2 / [1 / Sens + 1 / PPV]$$

In literal notation:

$$F = 2.TP / (2.TP + FP + FN)$$

In algebraic notation:

$$F = 2a / (2a + b + c)$$

F has range of 0 to 1, where 1 is perfect precision and recall [34].

**Worked Example: F Measure (F)**
In a screening test accuracy study of the MACE (N = 755) [16], at the cut-off giving maximal Youden index for dementia diagnosis, ≤20/30, TP = 104, FN =10, and FP = 188.
   Hence the value for F is:

$$F = 2.TP / (2.TP + FP + FN)$$
$$= (2 \times 104) / ([2 \times 104] + 188 + 10)$$
$$= 208 / 406$$
$$= 0.512$$

This may also be calculated using values of Sens = 0.912 (Sect. 2.2.1) and PPV = 0.356 (Sect. 2.3.1):

$$F = 2.PPV.Sens / (PPV + Sens)$$
$$= 2 \times 0.356 \times 0.912 / (0.356 + 0.912)$$
$$= 0.649 / 1.268$$
$$= 0.512$$

F measure ignores true negatives (TN or d), or correct "non-events", as does CSI (Sect. 4.8). There is a monotonic relation between the two measures, such that:

$$F = 2CSI / (1 + CSI)$$

Hence, when comparing different tests, the ranking is the same for F and CSI [15, 26] and the plot of F measure values against test cut-off [20] has the same maximum as for CSI and ETS (Fig. 4.7).

F measure has been calculated for several cognitive screening instruments [19] and varies with test cut-off or Q [20]. It also varies with prevalence: for the MACE study (Table 4.4; Fig. 4.8) the optimum value of F is at P = 0.7 (cf. Y and PSI). CSI would be anticipated to vary with P in the same manner.

**Table 4.4** Values of PPV (from Table 3.3), Sens (from Table 3.1), and F for dementia diagnosis at fixed MACE cut-off of ≤20/30 at various prevalence levels

| P, P′ | PPV | Sens | F |
|---|---|---|---|
| 0.1, 0.9 | 0.257 | 0.914 | 0.401 |
| 0.2, 0.8 | 0.437 | 0.908 | 0.590 |
| 0.3, 0.7 | 0.571 | 0.896 | 0.697 |
| 0.4, 0.6 | 0.675 | 0.884 | 0.765 |
| 0.5, 0.5 | 0.757 | 0.865 | 0.807 |
| 0.6, 0.4 | 0.824 | 0.840 | 0.832 |
| 0.7, 0.3 | 0.879 | 0.803 | 0.839 |
| 0.8, 0.2 | 0.926 | 0.746 | 0.826 |
| 0.9, 0.1 | 0.966 | 0.640 | 0.770 |

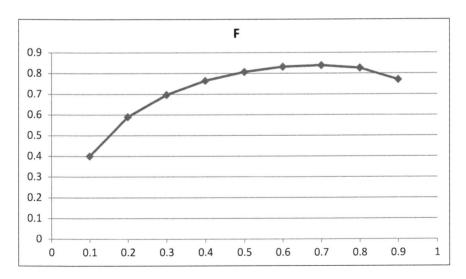

**Fig. 4.8** Plot of F (y axis) for dementia diagnosis at fixed Q (MACE cut-off ≤20/30) versus prevalence P (x axis)

F measure is a scalar value based on information from both columns of the $2 \times 2$ table (cf. Sens and Spec), hence varies with prevalence, P (Sect. 2.3.2), as well as with the level of the test, Q, and hence with test cut-off [20], and is also sensitive to class imbalance. Nevertheless, it has been advocated as a measure of agreement, using the nomenclature "proportion of specific positive agreement" (PA) [6], in preference to Cohen's kappa statistic (Sect. 7.2.2). Although the kappa statistic is often characterised as a measure of agreement, it is a relative measure and hence may be characterised as a measure of reliability. In this context, de Vet et al. [6] also characterised a "proportion of specific negative agreement" (NA):

$$
\begin{aligned}
NA &= 2.TN / (2TN + FP + FN) \\
&= 2d / (2d + b + c)
\end{aligned}
$$

Evidently this is equivalent to the harmonic mean of Spec and NPV:

$$
\begin{aligned}
NA &= 2.NPV.Spec / (NPV + Spec) \\
&= 2 / [1 / Spec + 1 / NPV]
\end{aligned}
$$

Thus, NA ignores true positives (TP or a), or "hits". It has a range of 0 to 1, where 1 is perfect NPV and specificity.

It is argued that these measures of specific agreement, PA and NA, facilitate clinical decision making in a way that relative measures such as Cohen's kappa do not [6].

---

**Worked Example: Proportion of Specific Negative Agreement (NA)**
In a screening test accuracy study of the MACE (N = 755) [16], at the cut-off giving maximal Youden index for dementia diagnosis, ≤20/30, FN =10, FP = 188, and TN = 453.
   Hence the value for NA is:

$$
\begin{aligned}
NA &= 2.TN / (2.TN + FP + FN) \\
&= (2 \times 453) / ([2 \times 453] + 188 + 10) \\
&= 906 / 1104 \\
&= 0.821
\end{aligned}
$$

This may also be calculated using values of Spec = 0.707 (Sect. 2.2.1) and NPV = 0.978 (Sect. 2.3.1):

$$
\begin{aligned}
NA &= 2.NPV.Spec / (NPV + Spec) \\
&= 2 \times 0.978 \times 0.707 / (0.978 + 0.707) \\
&= 1.383 / 1.685 \\
&= 0.821
\end{aligned}
$$

## 4.10   Summary Utility Index (SUI) and Summary Disutility Index (SDI)

A "summary utility index" (SUI) has been proposed [17, 21], based on the clinical utility indexes [30] (Sect. 2.4.2), defined as:

$$\begin{aligned} \mathrm{SUI} &= \left(\mathrm{CUI+} + \mathrm{CUI-}\right) \\ &= \left(\mathrm{Sens} \times \mathrm{PPV}\right) + \left(\mathrm{Spec} \times \mathrm{NPV}\right) \end{aligned}$$

SUI may thus range from 0 to 2, as for the "gain in certainty" [5] or overall correct classification rate [33] measure derived from Sens and Spec (see Sect. 3.2.5). SUI is therefore desirably as close to 2 as possible. It may be qualitatively classified, based on CUI values (Sect. 2.4.2), as: excellent $\geq 1.62$, good $\geq 1.28$, adequate $\geq 0.98$, poor $\geq 0.72$, or very poor $<0.72$ [17, 21].

In literal notation:

$$\begin{aligned} \mathrm{SUI} &= \left[\mathrm{TP}/\left(\mathrm{TP}+\mathrm{FN}\right) \times \mathrm{TP}/\left(\mathrm{TP}+\mathrm{FP}\right)\right] + \left[\mathrm{TN}/\left(\mathrm{FP}+\mathrm{TN}\right) \times \mathrm{TN}/\left(\mathrm{FN}+\mathrm{TN}\right)\right] \\ &= \mathrm{TP}^2/\left[\left(\mathrm{TP}+\mathrm{FN}\right)\left(\mathrm{TP}+\mathrm{FP}\right)\right] + \mathrm{TN}^2/\left[\left(\mathrm{FP}+\mathrm{TN}\right)\left(\mathrm{FN}+\mathrm{TN}\right)\right] \\ &= \mathrm{TP}^2/\left(\mathrm{p.q}\right) + \mathrm{TN}^2/\left(\mathrm{p'.q'}\right) \end{aligned}$$

In algebraic notation:

$$\begin{aligned} \mathrm{SUI} &= \left[a/\left(a+c\right) \times a/\left(a+b\right)\right] + \left[d/\left(b+d\right) \times d/\left(c+d\right)\right] \\ &= a^2/\left[\left(a+c\right).\left(a+b\right)\right] + d^2/\left[\left(b+d\right).\left(c+d\right)\right] \end{aligned}$$

and in terms of marginal totals:

$$\mathrm{SUI} = a^2/\left(\mathrm{p.q}\right) + d^2/\left(\mathrm{p'.q'}\right)$$

---

**Worked Example: Summary Utility Index (SUI)**
In a screening test accuracy study of MACE [16], at the MACE cut-off of $\leq 20/30$ for dementia diagnosis TP = 104, FN = 10, FP = 188, and TN = 453.
The values for Sens and Spec (Sect. 2.2.1) are:

$$\begin{aligned} \mathrm{Sens} &= 0.912 \\ \mathrm{Spec} &= 0.707 \end{aligned}$$

The values for PPV and NPV (Sect. 2.3.1) are:

$$\begin{aligned} \mathrm{PPV} &= 0.356 \\ \mathrm{NPV} &= 0.978 \end{aligned}$$

Hence the values for CUI+ and CUI- (Sect. 2.4.2) are:

$$
\begin{aligned}
\text{CUI+} &= \text{Sens} \times \text{PPV} \\
&= 0.912 \times 0.356 \\
&= 0.325
\end{aligned}
$$

$$
\begin{aligned}
\text{CUI-} &= \text{Spec} \times \text{NPV} \\
&= 0.707 \times 0.978 \\
&= 0.691
\end{aligned}
$$

Hence the value for SUI is:

$$
\begin{aligned}
\text{SUI} &= \text{CUI+} + \text{CUI-} \\
&= 0.325 + 0.691 \\
&= 1.016
\end{aligned}
$$

This value of SUI is qualitatively classified as adequate.

SUI values have been calculated for many neurological signs and cognitive screening questions and instruments [16, 17, 22–25]. SUI values vary with test cut-off or Q [16], with the same maximum as for other unitary metrics such as HMYPSI, MCC, CSI and F measure [20] (Table 6.2). SUI also varies with prevalence ([21], p.163–5).

SUI may be rescaled according to the level of the test, Q (see Sect. 2.2.2), such that [18]:

$$
\text{SUI}_Q = \text{CUI}_Q+ + \text{CUI}_Q-
$$

The reciprocal (multiplicative inverse) of SUI has been termed the number needed for screening utility (NNSU; Sect. 5.7) [17, 21].

A "summary disutility index" (SDI) may also be proposed based on the clinical disutility indexes (Sect. 2.4.2), defined as:

$$
\begin{aligned}
\text{SDI} &= \left( \text{CDI+} + \text{CDI-} \right) \\
&= \left( \text{FNR} \times \text{FDR} \right) + \left( \text{FPR} \times \text{FRR} \right)
\end{aligned}
$$

SDI may thus range from 0 to 2, as for SUI, and is desirably as close to 0 as possible. It may be qualitatively classified, based on CDI values (Sect. 2.4.2), as: very poor ≥1.62, poor ≥1.28, adequate ≥0.98, good ≥0.72, or excellent <0.72.

**Worked Example: Summary Disutility Index (SDI)**

In a screening test accuracy study of MACE [16], at the MACE cut-off of ≤20/30 for dementia diagnosis TP = 104, FN = 10, FP = 188, and TN = 453. The values for FNR and FPR (Sect. 2.2.3) are:

$$FNR = 0.088$$
$$FPR = 0.293$$

The values for FDR and FRR (Sect. 2.3.3) are:

$$FDR = 0.644$$
$$FRR = 0.022$$

Hence the values for CDI+ and CDI− (Sect. 2.4.2) are:

$$
\begin{aligned}
CDI+ &= FNR \times FDR \\
&= 0.088 \times 0.644 \\
&= 0.057
\end{aligned}
$$

$$
\begin{aligned}
CDI- &= FPR \times FRR \\
&= 0.293 \times 0.022 \\
&= 0.006
\end{aligned}
$$

Hence the value for SDI is:

$$
\begin{aligned}
SDI &= CDI+ + CDI- \\
&= 0.057 + 0.006 \\
&= 0.063
\end{aligned}
$$

This value of SDI is qualitatively classified as excellent.

# References

1. Boughorbel S, Jarray F, El-Anbari M. Optimal classifier for imbalanced data using Matthews Correlation Coefficient metric. PLoS One. 2017;12(6):e0177678.
2. Brenner H, Gefeller O. Variation of sensitivity, specificity, likelihood ratios and predictive values with disease prevalence. Stat Med. 1997;16:981–91.
3. Chicco D. Ten quick tips for machine learning in computational biology. BioData Min. 2017;10:35.
4. Chicco D, Jurman G. The advantages of the Matthews correlation coefficient (MCC) over F1 score and accuracy in binary classification evaluation. BMC Genomics. 2020;21:6.

5. Connell FA, Koepsell TD. Measures of gain in certainty from a diagnostic test. Am J Epidemiol. 1985;121:744–53.
6. De Vet HCW, Mokkink LB, Terwee CB, Hoekstra OS, Knol DL. Clinicians are right not to like Cohen's κ. BMJ. 2013;346:f2515.
7. Dice LR. Measures of the amount of ecological association between species. Ecology. 1945;26:297–302.
8. Doswell CA III, Davies-Jones R, Keller DL. On summary measures of skill in rare event forecasting based on contingency tables. Weather Forecast. 1990;5:576–85.
9. Gilbert GK. Finley's tornado predictions. Am Meteorol J. 1884;1:166–72.
10. Heston TF. Standardized predictive values. J Magn Reson Imaging. 2014;39:1338.
11. Hilden J, Glasziou P. Regret graphs, diagnostic uncertainty and Youden's index. Stat Med. 1996;15:969–86.
12. Hsieh S, McGrory S, Leslie F, Dawson K, Ahmed S, Butler CR, et al. The Mini-Addenbrooke's Cognitive Examination: a new assessment tool for dementia. Dement Geriatr Cogn Disord. 2015;39:1–11.
13. Hunink MGM, Weinstein MC, Wittenberg E, Drummond MF, Pliskin JS, Wong JB, et al. Decision making in health and medicine. Integrating evidence and values. 2nd ed. Cambridge: Cambridge University Press; 2014.
14. Jaccard P. The distribution of the flora in the alpine zone. New Phytologist. 1912;11:37–50.
15. Jolliffe IT. The Dice co-efficient: a neglected verification performance measure for deterministic forecasts of binary events. Meteorol Appl. 2016;23:89–90.
16. Larner AJ. MACE for diagnosis of dementia and MCI: examining cut-offs and predictive values. Diagnostics (Basel). 2019;9:E51.
17. Larner AJ. New unitary metrics for dementia test accuracy studies. Prog Neurol Psychiatry. 2019;23(3):21–5.
18. Larner AJ. Applying Kraemer's Q (positive sign rate): some implications for diagnostic test accuracy study results. Dement Geriatr Cogn Dis Extra. 2019;9:389–96.
19. Larner AJ. What is test accuracy? Comparing unitary accuracy metrics for cognitive screening instruments. Neurodegener Dis Manag. 2019;9:277–81.
20. Larner AJ. Defining "optimal" test cut-off using global test metrics: evidence from a cognitive screening instrument. Neurodegener Dis Manag. 2020;10:223–30.
21. Larner AJ. Manual of screeners for dementia: pragmatic test accuracy studies. London: Springer; 2020.
22. Larner AJ. Mini-Addenbrooke's Cognitive Examination (MACE): a useful cognitive screening instrument in older people? Can Geriatr J. 2020;23:199–204.
23. Larner AJ. Mini-Cog versus Codex (cognitive disorders examination): is there a difference? Dement Neuropsychol. 2020;14:128–33.
24. Larner AJ. Screening for dementia: Q* index as a global measure of test accuracy revisited. medRxiv. 2020; https://doi.org/10.1101/2020.04.01.20050567.
25. Larner AJ. The "attended alone" and "attended with" signs in the assessment of cognitive impairment: a revalidation. Postgrad Med. 2020;132:595–600.
26. Larner AJ. Assessing cognitive screening instruments with the critical success index. Prog Neurol Psychiatry. 2021;25(3):33–7.
27. Linn S, Grunau PD. New patient-oriented summary measure of net total gain in certainty for dichotomous diagnostic tests. Epidemiol Perspect Innov. 2006;3:11.
28. Matthews BW. Comparison of the predicted and observed secondary structure of T4 phage lysozyme. Biochem Biophys Acta. 1975;405:442–51.
29. Mitchell AJ. Index test. In: Kattan MW, editor. Encyclopedia of medical decision making. Los Angeles: Sage; 2009. p. 613–7.
30. Mitchell AJ. Sensitivity x PPV is a recognized test called the clinical utility index (CUI+). Eur J Epidemiol. 2011;26:251–2.
31. Palmer WC, Allen RA. Note on the accuracy of forecasts concerning the rain problem. U.S. Weather Bureau manuscript: Washington, DC; 1949.

32. Pencina MJ, D'Agostino RB Sr, D'Agostino RB Jr, Vasan RS. Evaluating the added predictive ability of a new marker: from area under the ROC curve to reclassification and beyond. Stat Med. 2008;27:157–72.
33. Perkins NJ, Schisterman EF. The inconsistency of "optimal" cutpoints obtained using two criteria based on the receiver operating characteristic curve. Am J Epidemiol. 2006;163:670–5.
34. Powers DMW. Evaluation: from precision, recall and F-measure to ROC, informedness, markedness and correlation. J Mach Learn Technol. 2011;2:37–63.
35. Powers DMW. What the F measure doesn't measure … Features, flaws, fallacies and fixes. arXiv. 2015; 1503.06410.2015.
36. Richard E, Schmand BA, Eikelenboom P, Van Gool WA. The Alzheimer's Disease Neuroimaging Initiative. MRI and cerebrospinal fluid biomarkers for predicting progression to Alzheimer's disease in patients with mild cognitive impairment: a diagnostic accuracy study. BMJ Open. 2013;3:e002541.
37. Schaefer JT. The critical success index as an indicator of warning skill. Weather Forecast. 1990;5:570–5.
38. Schisterman EF, Perkins NJ, Liu A, Bondell H. Optimal cut-point and its corresponding Youden Index to discriminate individuals using pooled blood samples. Epidemiology. 2005;16:73–81.
39. Smits N. A note on Youden's J and its cost ratio. BMC Med Res Methodol. 2010;10:89.
40. Sørensen T. A method of establishing groups of equal amplitude in plant sociology based on similarity of species and its application to analyses of the vegetation on Danish commons. K Dan Vidensk Sels. 1948;5:1–34.
41. Youden WJ. Index for rating diagnostic tests. Cancer. 1950;3:32–5.

# Chapter 5
# Reciprocal Measures

## Contents

## 5.1   Introduction

This chapter considers reciprocal or "number needed to" measures of test outcome which can be derived from the basic $2 \times 2$ contingency table, where reciprocal means multiplicative inverse [7, 12].

"Number needed to" measures were initially developed to summarise test impact in a manner deemed more intuitive to clinicians and patients than the traditional measures of discrimination such as sensitivity and specificity [17]. The "number needed to treat" (NNT) is a measure of therapeutic utility [3], equal to the reciprocal of absolute risk reduction, and the "number needed to harm" (NNH) is a measure of the adverse effects of therapeutic interventions [23]. Other adaptations of this method have also been made, such as the "number needed to see" for a specific event or occurrence to be encountered in clinical practice [6]. When "number needed" metrics refer to patients, it is obvious that only positive integer values are clinically meaningful, with absolute ("raw") values being rounded to the next highest integer value for purposes of clinical communication [8]. Although quite widely used as an outcome measure in therapeutic trials, NNT is recognised to have limitations, including the unspecified time frame of treatment, and the assumption that benefits are dichotomised rather than partial [21].

## 5.2   Number Needed to Diagnose (NND)

The reciprocal (multiplicative inverse) of the Youden index, Y (Sect. 4.2), has been defined by Linn and Grunau as the number needed to diagnose (NND) [18]. It may be expressed in terms of sensitivity (Sens) and specificity (Spec), and false positive (FPR) and false negative (FNR) rates (Sects. 2.2.1 and 2.2.3):

$$
\begin{aligned}
\mathrm{NND} \ &= \ 1/Y \\
&= \ 1/(\mathrm{Sens}+\mathrm{Spec}-1) \\
&= \ 1/\left[\mathrm{Sens}-(1-\mathrm{Spec})\right] \\
&= \ 1/(\mathrm{Sens}-\mathrm{FPR}) \\
&= \ 1/(\mathrm{TPR}-\mathrm{FPR}) \\
&= \ 1/\left[\mathrm{Spec}-(1-\mathrm{Sens})\right] \\
&= \ 1/(\mathrm{Spec}-\mathrm{FNR}) \\
&= \ 1/(\mathrm{TNR}-\mathrm{FNR}) \\
&= \ 1/\left[1-(\mathrm{FPR}+\mathrm{FNR})\right]
\end{aligned}
$$

As Y may also be expressed in terms of likelihood ratios (LRs) (Sect. 2.3.4) and correct classification and misclassification rates (Sect. 3.2.5), NND may also be expressed in these terms:

$$
\begin{aligned}
\mathrm{NND} \ &= \ 1/\left[(\mathrm{LR}+\ -1)\times(1-\mathrm{LR}-\ )/(\mathrm{LR}+\ -\ \mathrm{LR}-)\right] \\
&= \ (\mathrm{LR}+\ -\ \mathrm{LR}-)/\left[(\mathrm{LR}+\ -1)\times(1-\ \mathrm{LR}-)\right]
\end{aligned}
$$

$$
\begin{aligned}
\mathrm{NND} \ &= \ 1/(\mathrm{Correct\ classification\ rate}-1) \\
&= \ 1/(1-\mathrm{Misclassification\ rate})
\end{aligned}
$$

NND may be interpreted as the number of patients who need to be examined (for clinical signs) or tested (with a screening or diagnostic test) in order to detect correctly one person with the disease of interest in a study population of persons with and without the known disease.

In literal notation (see Fig. 1.1):

$$
\begin{aligned}
\mathrm{NND} \ &= \ 1/\left[\mathrm{TP}/(\mathrm{TP}+\mathrm{FN})+\mathrm{TN}/(\mathrm{FP}+\mathrm{TN})-1\right] \\
&= \ 1/\left[\mathrm{TP}/\mathrm{p}+\mathrm{TN}/\mathrm{p}'-1\right]
\end{aligned}
$$

In algebraic notation (see Fig. 1.2):

$$\begin{aligned} NND &= 1/\left[a/(a+c)+d/(b+d)-1\right] \\ &= (a+c).(b+d)/ad-bc \end{aligned}$$

In error notation (see Fig. 1.5):

$$NND = 1/\left[1-(\alpha+\beta)\right]$$

The range of Y is −1 to +1, so 1/Y could theoretically vary from −1 to +1. However, as the effective range of Y is 0 (no diagnostic value) to 1 (no false positives or false negatives), the anticipated range of 1/Y is ∞ (no diagnostic value) to 1 (no false positives or false negatives).

For diagnostic tests, low values of NND will therefore be desirable.

As the value of Y approaches 0, then NND values become inflated, as for any reciprocal (indeed if Y = 0, the division may be characterised as forbidden since it does not yield a unique result and is hence meaningless). This observation has prompted the opinion that NND is not a clinically meaningful number [19]. NND is also (notionally) insensitive to variation in disease prevalence, since it depends entirely on Sens and Spec [18]. This shortcoming may be addressed by using the number needed to predict (Sect. 5.3).

NND values vary with test cut-off [8].

**Worked Example: Number Needed to Diagnose (NND)**
The Mini-Addenbrooke's Cognitive Examination (MACE) [5] was subjected to a screening test accuracy study [8]. At the MACE cut-off of ≤20/30, the values for Sens and Spec (Sect. 2.2.1) were 0.912 and 0.707 respectively.

Hence the value for Y (Sect. 4.2) at this cut-off is:

$$\begin{aligned} Y &= Sens+Spec-1 \\ &= 0.912+0.707-1 \\ &= 0.619 \end{aligned}$$

The value for NND is:

$$\begin{aligned} NND &= 1/Y \\ &= 1/0.619 \\ &= 1.62 \end{aligned}$$

Referring to patients, NND is rounded up to the next whole integer and is therefore 2.

A rescaled NND may also be calculated [9]:

$$NND_Q \quad = \quad 1/Y_Q$$

## 5.3   Number Needed to Predict (NNP)

The reciprocal (multiplicative inverse) of the predictive summary index, PSI or $\Psi$ (Sect. 4.3), has been defined by Linn and Grunau as the number needed to predict (NNP) [18]. It may be expressed in terms of positive and negative predictive values (PPV, NPV), and false discovery (FDR) and false reassurance (FRR) rates (Sects. 2.3.1 and 2.3.3):

$$
\begin{aligned}
NNP \quad &= \quad 1/PSI \\
&= \quad 1/(PPV + NPV - 1) \\
&= \quad 1/\left[PPV - (1 - NPV)\right] \\
&= \quad 1/(PPV - FRR) \\
&= \quad 1/\left[NPV - (1 - PPV)\right] \\
&= \quad 1/(NPV - FDR)
\end{aligned}
$$

NNP may be interpreted as the number of patients who need to be examined or tested in the patient population in order to predict correctly the diagnosis of one person.

In literal notation:

$$
\begin{aligned}
NNP \quad &= \quad 1/\left[TP/(TP + FP) + TN/(FN + TN) - 1\right] \\
&= \quad 1/\left[TP/q + TN/q' - 1\right]
\end{aligned}
$$

In algebraic notation:

$$
\begin{aligned}
NNP \quad &= \quad 1/\left[a/(a + b) + d/(c + d) - 1\right] \\
&= \quad (a + b).(c + d)/(ad - bc)
\end{aligned}
$$

As the effective range of PSI is 0 (no diagnostic value) to 1 (no false positives or false negatives), the anticipated range of 1/PSI is $\infty$ (no diagnostic value) to 1 (no false positives or false negatives). For diagnostic tests, low values of NNP will therefore be desirable. NNP is dependent on disease prevalence and is therefore deemed a better descriptor of diagnostic tests than NND in patient populations with different prevalence of disease [18].

NNP values vary with test cut-off [8].

**Worked Example: Number Needed to Predict (NNP)**
In a screening test accuracy study of MACE [8], at the MACE cut-off of
≤20/30, the values for PPV and NPV (Sect. 2.3.1) were 0.356 and 0.978
respectively.
Hence the value for PSI (Sect. 4.3) at this cut-off is:

$$
\begin{aligned}
\text{PSI} &= \text{PPV} + \text{NPV} - 1 \\
&= 0.356 + 0.978 - 1 \\
&= 0.334
\end{aligned}
$$

The value for NNP is:

$$
\begin{aligned}
\text{NNP} &= 1/\text{PSI} \\
&= 1/0.334 \\
&= 2.99
\end{aligned}
$$

Referring to patients, NND is rounded up to the next whole integer and is
therefore 3.

## 5.4  Number Needed to Misdiagnose (NNM)

The reciprocal (multiplicative inverse) of inaccuracy (Sect. 3.2.4) has been defined
as the "number needed to misdiagnose" (NNM) [4]:

$$
\begin{aligned}
\text{NNM} &= 1/\text{Inaccuracy} \\
&= 1/(1-\text{Accuracy})
\end{aligned}
$$

In literal notation:

$$
\begin{aligned}
\text{NNM} &= 1/\left[(FP+FN)/(TP+FP+FN+TN)\right] \\
&= 1/\left[(FP+FN)/N\right] \\
&= N/(FP+FN)
\end{aligned}
$$

In algebraic notation:

$$
\begin{aligned}
\text{NNM} &= 1/\left[(b+c)/(a+b+c+d)\right] \\
&= 1/\left[(b+c)/N\right] \\
&= N/(b+c)
\end{aligned}
$$

NNM is characterised as a measure of effectiveness, the number of patients who need to be examined or tested in order for one to be misdiagnosed [4]. For diagnostic tests, high values of NNM will therefore be desirable.

NNM values vary with test cut-off [8].

---

**Worked Example: Number Needed to Misdiagnose (NNM)**

In a screening test accuracy study of MACE [8], at the MACE cut-off of ≤20/30, the values for Acc and Inacc (Sect. 3.2.4) were 0.738 and 0.262 respectively.

Hence the value for NNM at this cut-off is:

$$
\begin{aligned}
NNM &= 1/\text{Inaccuracy} \\
&= 1/(1-\text{Accuracy}) \\
&= 1/0.262 \\
&= 3.82
\end{aligned}
$$

Alternatively, at this cut-off in the MACE study (N = 755), FN = 10 and FP = 188 (Fig. 2.2).

$$
\begin{aligned}
NNM &= N/(FP+FN) \\
&= 755/(188+10) \\
&= 3.81
\end{aligned}
$$

[The different results relate to rounding errors.]

Referring to patients, NNM is rounded up to the next whole integer and is therefore 4.

---

## 5.5  Likelihood to Be Diagnosed or Misdiagnosed (LDM)

Consideration of the numbers needed to diagnose (NND; Sect. 5.2), predict (NNP; Sect. 5.3), and misdiagnose (NNM; Sect. 5.4) prompts the inclusion here of the likelihood to diagnose or misdiagnose (LDM) parameter, even though it is not a reciprocal measure, since it is intimately related to these reciprocal measures [10, 12].

The "number needed" metrics used to describe therapeutic studies, NNT and NNH (Sect. 5.1), were combined by Citrome and Ketter [2] to produce a "likelihood to be helped or harmed" (LHH) metric to summarise the effects of a therapeutic intervention:

$$\text{LHH} \quad = \quad \text{NNH}\,/\,\text{NNT}$$

LHH values are ideally as large as possible, since NNH is desirably large and NNT is desirably small. LHH values are reported to help clinicians and patients to evaluate potential risk-benefit trade-offs of treatment [1].

The "likelihood to be diagnosed or misdiagnosed" (LDM) [7, 8, 10, 11] was developed as analogous to LHH but for use in test accuracy studies. Two formulations of LDM were formulated:

$$\text{LDM} \quad = \quad \text{NNM}\,/\,\text{NND}$$

and:

$$\text{LDM} \quad = \quad \text{NNM}\,/\,\text{NNP}$$

The latter might also be termed the "likelihood to be predicted or misdiagnosed" (LPM) to distinguish it from the other formulation.

For LDM = NNM/NND:

$$\text{LDM} \quad = \quad \left[1/(1-\text{Acc})\right]/(1/\text{Y})$$
$$= \quad \text{Y}\,/\,\text{Inacc}$$

In literal notation:

$$\text{LDM} = \left(1/\left[(\text{FP}+\text{FN})/(\text{TP}+\text{FP}+\text{FN}+\text{TN})\right]\right)/\left(1/\left[\text{TP}/(\text{TP}+\text{FN})+\text{TN}/(\text{FP}+\text{TN})-1\right]\right)$$
$$= \left(1/\left[(\text{FP}+\text{FN})/(\text{TP}+\text{FP}+\text{FN}+\text{TN})\right]\right)/\left(1/\left[\text{TP}/(\text{TP}+\text{FN})-\text{FP}/(\text{FP}+\text{TN})\right]\right)$$
$$= \left[\text{TP}/(\text{TP}+\text{FN})-\text{FP}/(\text{FP}+\text{TN})\right]/\left[(\text{FP}+\text{FN})\right]/(\text{TP}+\text{FP}+\text{FN}+\text{TN})$$

In algebraic notation:

$$\text{LDM} \quad = \quad \left(1/\left[(b+c)/(a+b+c+d)\right]\right)/\left(1/\left[a/(a+c)+d/(b+d)-1\right]\right)$$
$$= \quad \left(1/\left[(b+c)/(a+b+c+d)\right]\right)/\left(1/\left[a/(a+c)-b/(b+d)\right]\right)$$
$$= \quad \left[a/(a+c)-b/(b+d)\right]/\left[(b+c)/(a+b+c+d)\right]$$

A rescaled form may also be calculated for this variant of LDM [9]:

$$\text{LDM}_Q \quad = \quad \text{NNM}\,/\,\text{NND}_Q$$

For the likelihood to be predicted or misdiagnosed:

$$\text{LPM} \quad = \quad \text{NNM}\,/\,\text{NNP}$$
$$= \quad \left[1/(1-\text{Acc})\right]/(1/\text{PSI})$$
$$= \quad \text{PSI}\,/\,\text{Inacc}$$

**Worked Examples: Likelihood to Be Diagnosed or Misdiagnosed (LDM)**
In a screening test accuracy study of MACE [8], at the MACE cut-off of
≤20/30, the absolute ("raw") values for NND (Sect. 5.2) and NNM (Sect. 5.4)
were 1.62 and 3.82 respectively.
Hence the value for LDM at this cut-off is:

$$\begin{aligned} LDM &= NNM/NND \\ &= 3.82/1.62 \\ &= 2.36 \end{aligned}$$

LDM may also be calculated from the values of Y (Sect. 4.2) and Inacc
(Sect. 3.2.4), as:

$$\begin{aligned} LDM &= Y/Inacc \\ &= 0.619/0.262 \\ &= 2.36 \end{aligned}$$

In literal notation:

$$\begin{aligned} LDM &= 1/\left[(FP+FN)/(TP+FP+FN+TN)\right]/\left(1/\left[TP/(TP+FP)+TN/(FN+TN)-1\right]\right) \\ &= 1/\left[(FP+FN)/(TP+FP+FN+TN)\right]/\left(1/\left[TP/(TP+FP)-FN/(FN+TN)\right]\right) \\ &= \left[TP/(TP+FP)-FN/(FN+TN)\right]/\left[(FP+FN)/(TP+FP+FN+TN)\right] \end{aligned}$$

In algebraic notation:

$$\begin{aligned} LPM &= \left(1/\left[(b+c)/(a+b+c+d)\right]\right)/\left(1/\left[a/(a+b)+d/(c+d)-1\right]\right) \\ &= \left(1/\left[(b+c)/(a+b+c+d)\right]\right)/\left(1/\left[a/(a+b)-c/(c+d)\right]\right) \\ &= \left[a/(a+b)-c/(c+d)\right]/\left[(b+c)/(a+b+c+d)\right] \end{aligned}$$

Hence LDM and LPM may be conceptualised as ratios of benefits (correct diagnosis, correct prediction) and harms (misdiagnosis). These may be compared with
the net harm to net benefit (H/B) ratio (see Sect. 2.3.5). LDM and LPM values vary
with test cut-off [8], and plotting these shows maxima similar to many of the other
unitary tests considered in Chap. 4 (Fig. 5.1; Table 6.2).
Both LDM and LPM have a range of −1 (Y or PSI = −1, Inacc = 1) to ∞ (Y or
PSI = +1, Inacc = 0). Since for diagnostic tests low values of NND and NNP and

**Worked Examples: Likelihood to Be Predicted or Misdiagnosed (LPM)**
In a screening test accuracy study of MACE [8], at the MACE cut-off of
≤20/30, the absolute ("raw") values for NNP (Sect. 5.3) and NNM (Sect. 5.4)
are 2.99, and 3.82 respectively.
Hence the value for LPM at this cut-off is:

$$
\begin{aligned}
LPM &= NNM / NNP \\
&= 3.82 / 2.99 \\
&= 1.28
\end{aligned}
$$

LPM may also be calculated from the values of PSI (Sect. 4.3) and Inacc
(Sect. 3.2.4), as:

$$
\begin{aligned}
LPM &= PSI / Inacc \\
&= 0.334 / 0.262 \\
&= 1.27
\end{aligned}
$$

[The different results relate to rounding errors.]

high values of NNM are desirable, higher values of LDM and LPM (>1) would suggest a test more likely to favour correct diagnosis or prediction over misdiagnosis,
whereas lower values of LDM and LPM (<1) suggest misdiagnosis is more likely
than correct diagnosis or prediction. LDM values as high as ~7 have been recorded
for tests which are both highly sensitive and specific ( [12], p.75).

LDM and LPM should help clinicians and patients to evaluate potential risk-
benefit trade-offs with particular diagnostic tests, and hence inform clinical decision
making. For example, testing positive on a test with high LDM may permit a confi-
dent diagnosis, unlike the situation with a low LDM test, indeed the latter might be
avoided for this very reason, especially if the test is expensive and/or poses risks to
the patient.

The LDM formulations have found application in the evaluation of individual
neurological signs and cognitive screening instruments [7, 8, 10–16, 24, 25] and
also using data from meta-analyses of cognitive screening instruments [22,
24]. Other methods to calculate a "likelihood to be diagnosed or misdiagnosed" are
currently in development (Larner, submitted).

**Fig. 5.1** Plot of likelihood to be diagnosed or misdiagnosed (LDM; diamonds) and likelihood to be predicted or misdiagnosed (LPM; triangles) on the y axis versus MACE cut-off (x axis). (Adapted from [13])

## 5.6  Number Needed to Screen (NNS)

A "number needed to screen" (NNS) metric was first defined for use in public health epidemiology, defined as the number of people that need to be screened for a given duration to prevent one death or adverse event [20].

In terms of screening or diagnostic test accuracy studies, a "number needed to screen" (NNS) metric has been defined as the number of patients who need to be screened in order for one additional correct identification beyond those misidentified [19]. NNS is derived from the identification index (II) (Sect. 4.6):

$$
\begin{aligned}
\mathrm{NNS} \; &= \; 1/\,\mathrm{II} \\
&= \; 1/\big[\,\mathrm{Acc} - \big(\mathrm{Inacc}\big)\big] \\
&= \; 1/\big[\,\mathrm{Acc} - \big(1 - \mathrm{Acc}\big)\big] \\
&= \; 1/\big(2.\mathrm{Acc} - 1\big)
\end{aligned}
$$

II ranges from −1 to +1 (Sect. 4.6), as for Y and PSI. However, whereas negative values are not anticipated with Y and PSI, any value of Acc <0.5 (i.e. Inacc >0.5) will result in a negative value of II, and hence a negative value of NNS. As only positive integer values are clinically meaningful for "number needed" metrics when these refer to patients, negative NNS values are clinically meaningless.

In literal notation:

$$NNS = 1/\left[2.(TP+TN)/(TP+FP+FN+TN)-1\right]$$
$$= 1/\left[2.(TP+TN)/N-1\right]$$

In algebraic notation:

$$NNS = 1/\left[2.(a+d)/(a+b+c+d)-1\right]$$
$$= 1/\left[2.(a+d)/N-1\right]$$

NNS varies with test cut-off [8].

**Worked Example: Number Needed to Screen (NNS)**
In a screening test accuracy study of MACE [8], at the MACE cut-off of $\leq$20/30, TP = 104, FN =10, FP = 188, and TN = 453 (Fig. 2.2).
   The value for Acc (Sect. 3.2.4) is:

$$Acc = (TP+TN)/(TP+FN+FP+TN)$$
$$= (104+453)/(104+10+188+453)$$
$$= 0.738$$

The value for II (Sect. 4.6) is:

$$II = 2.Acc-1$$
$$= (2\times0.738)-1$$
$$= 0.475$$

Hence, the value for NNS is:

$$NNS = 1/(2.Acc-1)$$
$$= 1/0.475$$
$$= 2.11$$

   Referring to patients, NNS is rounded up to the next whole integer and is therefore 3.

## 5.7  Number Needed for Screening Utility (NNSU) and Number Needed for Screening Disutility (NNSD)

The number needed for screening utility (NNSU) is the reciprocal or multiplicative inverse of SUI (Sect. 4.10) [10, 12]:

$$
\begin{aligned}
\text{NNSU} &= 1/\text{SUI} \\
&= 1/\left(\text{CUI+} + \text{CUI-}\right) \\
&= 1/\left(\text{Sens} \times \text{PPV}\right) + \left(\text{Spec} \times \text{NPV}\right)
\end{aligned}
$$

SUI ranges from 0 to 2 (Sect. 4.10). Hence NNSU ranges from $\infty$ (SUI = 0, no screening value) to 0.5 (SUI = 2, perfect screening utility), with low values of NNSU desirable. All NNSU values are positive (cf. NNS, Sect. 5.6). Following the qualitative classification of SUI (Sect. 4.10), it is also possible to classify NNSU values qualitatively. Generally, NNSU values may be dichotomised, as <1 being acceptable or desirable, >1 not so ("inadequate") [10, 12].

In literal notation:

$$
\begin{aligned}
\text{NNSU} &= 1/\text{TP}^2/\left[\left(\text{TP}+\text{FN}\right)\left(\text{TP}+\text{FP}\right)\right] + \text{TN}^2/\left[\left(\text{TN}+\text{FP}\right)\left(\text{TN}+\text{FN}\right)\right] \\
&= 1/\left[\text{TP}^2/\text{p.q}\right] + \left[\text{TN}^2/\text{p'.q'}\right]
\end{aligned}
$$

In algebraic notation:

$$
\begin{aligned}
\text{NNSU} &= 1/\left[a/\left(a+c\right) \times a/\left(a+b\right) + d/\left(b+d\right) \times d/\left(c+d\right)\right] \\
&= 1/a^2/\left[\left(a+c\right).\left(a+b\right)\right] + d^2/\left[\left(b+d\right).\left(c+d\right)\right]
\end{aligned}
$$

A rescaled form may also be calculated [9]:

$$
\text{NNSU}_Q = 1/\text{SUI}_Q
$$

NNSU values vary with test cut-off [8].

**Worked Example: Number Needed for Screening Utility (NNSU)**
In a screening test accuracy study of MACE [8], at the MACE cut-off of
$\leq$20/30, CUI+ = 0.325 and CUI− = 0.691 (Sect. 2.4.2).
Hence the value for SUI (Sect. 4.10) is:

$$
\begin{aligned}
\text{SUI} \; &= \; \text{CUI+} + \text{CUI−} \\
&= \; 0.325 + 0.691 \\
&= \; 1.016
\end{aligned}
$$

The value for NNSU is:

$$
\begin{aligned}
\text{NNSU} \; &= \; 1/\text{SUI} \\
&= \; 1/1.016 \\
&= \; 0.984
\end{aligned}
$$

This value of NNSU is qualitatively classified as adequate. As it refers to
patients, NNSU is rounded up to the next whole integer and is therefore 1.

NNSU values have been calculated for many neurological signs and cognitive
screening questions and instruments [8, 10, 12, 14–16].

The number needed for screening disutility (NNSD) is the reciprocal or multiplicative inverse of SDI (Sect. 4.10):

$$
\begin{aligned}
\text{NNSD} \; &= \; 1/\text{SDI} \\
&= \; 1/(\text{CDI+} + \text{CDI−}) \\
&= \; 1/\left[(\text{FNR} \times \text{FDR}) + (\text{FPR} \times \text{FRR})\right]
\end{aligned}
$$

SDI ranges from 0 to 2 (Sect. 4.10). Hence NNSD ranges from $\infty$ (SDI = 0, no
screening disutility) to 0.5 (SDI = 2, maximum screening disutility), with high values of NNSD desirable. Generally, as for NNSU, NNSD values may be dichotomised, as >1 being acceptable or desirable, <1 not so.

**Worked Example: Number Needed for Screening Disutility (NNSD)**
In a screening test accuracy study of MACE [8], at the MACE cut-off of
$\leq20/30$, CDI+ = 0.057 and CDI− = 0.006 (Sect. 2.4.2).
Hence the value for SDI (Sect. 4.10) is:

$$
\begin{aligned}
SDI &= CDI{+} + CDI{-} \\
&= 0.057 + 0.006 \\
&= 0.063
\end{aligned}
$$

The value for NNSD is:

$$
\begin{aligned}
NNSD &= 1/SDI \\
&= 1/0.063 \\
&= 15.87
\end{aligned}
$$

This value of NNSD is qualitatively classified as adequate. As it refers to
patients, NNSD is rounded up to the next whole integer and is therefore 16.

# References

1. Andrade C. Likelihood of being helped or harmed as a measure of clinical outcomes in psychopharmacology. J Clin Psychiatry. 2017;78:e73–5.
2. Citrome L, Ketter TA. When does a difference make a difference? Interpretation of number needed to treat, number needed to harm, and likelihood to be helped or harmed. Int J Clin Pract. 2013;67:407–11.
3. Cook RJ, Sackett DL. The number needed to treat: a clinically useful measure of treatment effect. BMJ. 1995;310:452–4.
4. Habibzadeh F, Yadollahie M. Number needed to misdiagnose: a measure of diagnostic test effectiveness. Epidemiology. 2013;24:170.
5. Hsieh S, McGrory S, Leslie F, Dawson K, Ahmed S, Butler CR, et al. The Mini-Addenbrooke's Cognitive Examination: a new assessment tool for dementia. Dement Geriatr Cogn Disord. 2015;39:1–11.
6. Larner AJ. Teleneurology by internet and telephone. A study of medical self-help. London: Springer; 2011.
7. Larner AJ. Number needed to diagnose, predict, or misdiagnose: useful metrics for non-canonical signs of cognitive status? Dement Geriatr Cogn Dis Extra. 2018;8:321–7.
8. Larner AJ. MACE for diagnosis of dementia and MCI: examining cut-offs and predictive values. Diagnostics (Basel). 2019;9:E51.
9. Larner AJ. Applying Kraemer's Q (positive sign rate): some implications for diagnostic test accuracy study results. Dement Geriatr Cogn Dis Extra. 2019;9:389–96.
10. Larner AJ. New unitary metrics for dementia test accuracy studies. Prog Neurol Psychiatry. 2019;23(3):21–5.

11. Larner AJ. Evaluating cognitive screening instruments with the "likelihood to be diagnosed or misdiagnosed" measure. Int J Clin Pract. 2019;73:e13265.
12. Larner AJ. Manual of screeners for dementia: pragmatic test accuracy studies. London: Springer; 2020.
13. Larner AJ. Defining "optimal" test cut-off using global test metrics: evidence from a cognitive screening instrument. Neurodegener Dis Manag. 2020;10:223–30.
14. Larner AJ. Mini-Addenbrooke's Cognitive Examination (MACE): a useful cognitive screening instrument in older people? Can Geriatr J. 2020;23:199–204.
15. Larner AJ. Mini-Cog versus Codex (cognitive disorders examination): is there a difference? Dement Neuropsychol. 2020;14:128–33.
16. Larner AJ. The "attended alone" and "attended with" signs in the assessment of cognitive impairment: a revalidation. Postgrad Med. 2020;132:595–600.
17. Laupacis A, Sackett DL, Roberts RS. An assessment of clinically useful measures of the consequences of treatment. N Engl J Med. 1988;318:1728–33.
18. Linn S, Grunau PD. New patient-oriented summary measure of net total gain in certainty for dichotomous diagnostic tests. Epidemiol Perspect Innov. 2006;3:11.
19. Mitchell AJ. Index test. In: Kattan MW, editor. Encyclopedia of medical decision making. Los Angeles: Sage; 2009. p. 613–7.
20. Rembold CM. Number needed to screen: development of a statistic for disease screening. BMJ. 1998;317:307–12.
21. Wald NJ, Morris JK. Two under-recognized limitations of number needed to treat. Int J Epidemiol. 2020;49:359–60.
22. Williamson JC, Larner AJ. "Likelihood to be diagnosed or misdiagnosed": application to meta-analytic data for cognitive screening instruments. Neurodegener Dis Manag. 2019;9:91–5.
23. Zermansky A. Number needed to harm should be measured for treatments. BMJ. 1998;317:1014.
24. Ziso B, Larner AJ. AD8: Likelihood to diagnose or misdiagnose. J Neurol Neurosurg Psychiatry. 2019;90:A20. (https://jnnp.bmj.com/content/90/12/A20.1)
25. Ziso B, Larner AJ. Codex (cognitive disorders examination) decision tree modified for the detection of dementia and MCI. Diagnostics (Basel). 2019;9:E58.

# Chapter 6
# Measures Not Directly Related to the 2 × 2 Contingency Table

## Contents

## 6.1 Introduction

The methods of analysis of 2 × 2 contingency tables considered in the previous chapters of this book have all been arithmetical or algebraic. Graphical depiction of test performance is also possible, and the core content of this chapter. One of these performance graphing methods, the receiver operating characteristic (ROC) curve or plot, is also relevant to the definition of "optimal" test cut-offs which may in turn be used to calibrate test results when constructing 2 × 2 contingency tables (Sect. 1.5).

© Springer Nature Switzerland AG 2021

A. J. Larner, *The 2x2 Matrix*, https://doi.org/10.1007/978-3-030-74920-0_6

## 6.2   Receiver Operating Characteristic (ROC) Plot or Curve

The receiver operating characteristic (ROC) curve or plot is a frequently used method to display the cumulated results of a quantitative test accuracy study [11, 24, 57, 59], which takes its origins in signal detection theory [38, 39]. In unit 2-dimensional ROC space, the Sensitivity (Sens), or "hit rate" or true positive rate (TPR), of the test is plotted on the ordinate against false positive rate (FPR), the complement of Specificity (Spec), or (1 – Specificity), on the abscissa across the range of possible test scores with linear interpolation between points (an example is shown in Fig. 6.1 [28]). Empirically, this is a step function, tending to a curve as the number of instances, and hence points, approaches infinity.

(Sometimes authors reverse the direction of the x-axis on the ROC plot, such that the origin coordinates become (1,0), and the abscissa thus plots specificity.)

The ROC plot is a graph of the relative trade-off of benefits, TPR (Sect. 2.2.1), against costs, FPR (Sect. 2.2.3), extending from conservative cut-offs (bottom left, coordinates (0,0), Sens = 0, Spec = 1) to liberal cut-offs (top right, coordinates (1,1), Sens = 1, Spec = 0). ROC plots ideally approximate the top left hand ("north west") corner of the ROC space (coordinates (0,1), Sens = 1, Spec = 1), corresponding to isosensitivity. In the situation where false positive rates are very low, it has been questioned whether ROC plotting is profitable ([55], p. 153).

ROC curves may be described as "threshold agnostic" or "threshold free", since test performance is shown without a specific threshold. ROC curves may also be used to define an optimal threshold (methods discussed below, Sects. 6.2.1, 6.2.2, 6.2.3, and 6.2.4). Moreover, as TPR and FPR are strict columnar ratios, algebraically independent of base rate, the ROC plot is insensitive to changes in class distribution.

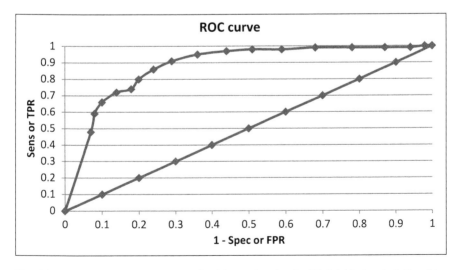

**Fig. 6.1** Empirical ROC plot for diagnosis of dementia using the Mini-Addenbrooke's Cognitive Examination (MACE), with chance diagonal (y = x). (Modified from [28]). TPR true positive rate, FPR false positive rate

ROC plots typically include the diagonal 45° line through ROC space (y = x, or Sens = 1 – Spec, or TPR = FPR) which represents the performance of a random classifier or the chance level (Fig. 6.1). This line also corresponds to a diagnostic odds ratio (DOR) = 1, indicative of a useless test, and reflective of the relationship between DOR and Sens and Spec (Sect. 2.4.1). ROC curves which are symmetrical with respect to the anti-diagonal line through ROC space (y = 1 – x) have a constant DOR (isocontours, which might be termed "isoDORs"), with DOR value varying from ∞ in the optimal ("north west") plot, running through coordinates (0,1) with y = 1 at the intersection with the ROC anti-diagonal, to –∞ at the bottom right hand ("south east") corner, running through coordinates (1,0) with y = 0 at the intersection with the ROC anti-diagonal.

The slope of a tangent to the ROC curve at any point is equal to the likelihood ratio (= TPR/FPR; Sect. 2.3.4) at that point [3], but the step function nature of most ROC plots makes it difficult to identify the point of maximum slope [13]. The slope is also related to the net harm to net benefit (H/B) ratio (Sects. 2.3.5 and 3.2.5), since:

$$
\begin{aligned}
\mathrm{Net\,Harm}(H) / \mathrm{Net\,Benefit}(B) &= \text{Pre-test odds} \times \mathrm{LR+} \\
&= (P/P') \times \mathrm{LR+} \\
&= (P/P') \times (\mathrm{TPR/FPR})
\end{aligned}
$$

and:

$$
\mathrm{Net\,Harm}(H) / \mathrm{Net\,Benefit}(B) = C_{FP} - C_{TN} / C_{FN} - C_{TP}
$$

Combining:

$$
\begin{aligned}
C_{FP} - C_{TN} / C_{FN} - C_{TP} &= \text{Pre-test odds} \times \mathrm{LR+}\ \text{Pre-test odds} \times \mathrm{LR+} \\
&= (P/P') \times \mathrm{LR+} \\
&= (P/P') \times (\mathrm{TPR/FPR})
\end{aligned}
$$

and rearranging:

$$
\begin{aligned}
\mathrm{LR+} = \mathrm{TPR/FPR} &= (C_{FP} - C_{TN} / C_{FN} - C_{TP}) \times (P'/P) \\
&= H/B \times (P'/P)
\end{aligned}
$$

The area under the ROC curve (AUC) is the probability that a random person with disease has a value of the measurement above the cut-off compared to a random person without disease, or the percentage correct in a two-alternative forced choice task. This scalar value, also referred to as the concordance statistic or c-statistc, represents expected test performance and hence may be used as a measure of diagnostic accuracy (cf. other meanings of "accuracy", Sect. 3.2.4 [29]). The performance of a random classifier gives AUC ROC = 0.5; confidence intervals of AUC overlapping this value suggest the null hypothesis cannot be rejected. AUC <0.5 is an outcome worse than random guessing. Various qualitative classification

**Table 6.1** Classifications of ROC plot AUC values

| Metz [42] (1978): |
| --- |
| • between 0.9–1.0: excellent |
| • 0.8–0.9: good |
| • 0.7–0.8: fair |
| • 0.6–0.7: poor |
| • 0.5–0.6: failed |
| Swets [53] (1988): |
| • ≥0.91: high accuracy |
| • 0.71–0.90: moderate accuracy |
| • 0.50–0.70: low accuracy |
| Jones and Athanasiou [21] (2005): |
| • ≥0.97: excellent |
| • 0.93–0.96: very good |
| • 0.75–0.92: good |

schemata for AUC values have been reported (Table 6.1) [21, 42, 53]. AUC values tend to be optimistic compared to other accuracy measures [29].

Methods for calculation of AUC are mainly based on a non-parametric statistical test, the Wilcoxon rank-sum test, namely the proportion of all possible pairs of non-diseased and diseased test subjects for which the diseased result is higher than the

**Worked Example: AUC ROC Plot**
The Mini-Addenbrooke's Cognitive Examination (MACE) [18], a brief cognitive screening instrument, was subjected to a screening test accuracy study in a large patient cohort, N = 755 [28]. From a ROC plot of the results (Fig. 6.1), AUC was calculated by rank-sum methods as AUC = 0.886, a value which may be qualitatively categorised as good [21, 42] or moderate [53].

The MACE ROC plot is asymmetric (Fig. 6.1), so DOR varies with test cut-off, with a maximal value of 52.8 at MACE cut-off of ≤23/30 [31]. AUC was calculated, at this maximal DOR [30], as [54]:

$$
\begin{aligned}
\mathrm{AUC} &= \mathrm{DOR}/(\mathrm{DOR}-1)^2 \cdot \left[(\mathrm{DOR}-1) - \log_e(\mathrm{DOR})\right] \\
&= 0.0197 \times 47.833 \\
&= 0.941
\end{aligned}
$$

This is greater than the AUC value by rank-sum methods (0.886), presumably because the equation assumes a symmetric ROC curve with DOR = 52.8. The DOR-based AUC value may be qualitatively categorised as excellent [42], very good [21], or high accuracy [53]. Hence the categorisation of AUC has changed according to method of its calculation.

non-diseased plus half the proportion of ties [9, 15, 16, 59, 60]. AUC may also be calculated from the DOR using the formula [54]:

$$AUC = DOR / (DOR - 1)^2 . [(DOR - 1) - \log_e (DOR)]$$

The latter may tend to overestimate AUC compared to the rank-sum method [30, 41].

ROC plots have some shortcomings. The combination of test accuracy over a range of thresholds includes those which may be both clinically relevant and clinically nonsensical [40]. Hence only parts of ROC plots may be of clinical interest. Methods for partial ROC curve analysis are available [58]. A ROC plot may also be divided graphically to illustrate zones of test efficacy, the so-called zombie ("zones of mostly bad imaging efficacy") plot [48], although the technique is applicable to diagnostic tests other than imaging.

For a categorical classifier with n thresholds, there will be (n − 1) points in ROC space. Hence classifiers with a binary outcome produce a ROC dot rather than plot, and an area under a triangle rather than an area under a curve (Fig. 6.2). For the particular case of a binary classifier, it has been shown that the value of AUC also simplifies [44], to:

$$AUC \quad = \quad \frac{1}{2}.(Sens + Spec)$$

This corresponds to "balanced accuracy" defined as (Sens + Spec)/2.
This may also be expressed in terms of the Youden index, Y (Sect. 4.2):

$$Y \quad = \quad Sens + Spec - 1$$
$$Y + 1 \quad = \quad Sens + Spec$$

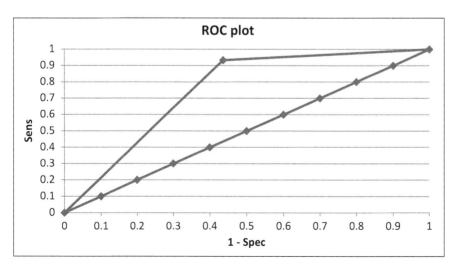

**Fig. 6.2** ROC plot for a binary classifier: attended alone/attended with sign for the diagnosis of any cognitive impairment (dementia + MCI) versus no cognitive impairment, with chance diagonal (y = x). (Data from [32], plot adapted from [41])

Substituting:

$$AUC = \tfrac{1}{2}.(Y+1)$$

or:

$$Y = 2.AUC-1$$

Whether ROC plots can be meaningfully applied in the assessment of binary categorical tests remains moot [41, 44].

One of the key functions of ROC plots is to permit the definition of "optimal" test cut-offs (Sect. 1.6). Other methods for defining optimal cut-offs independent of the ROC plot are also available. These various approaches are now considered.

**Worked Example: AUC ROC Plot for Single Fixed Threshold**

If MACE is treated as a binary classifier with a single fixed threshold of ≤20/30 (based on maximal Youden index; Sect. 4.2), as shown in Fig. 6.3, AUC by rank-sum methods = 0.809. This may also be calculated from Sens = 0.912 and Spec = 0.707 at this MACE cut-off (Sect. 2.2.1):

$$\begin{aligned} AUC &= \tfrac{1}{2}.(Sens+Spec) \\ &= \tfrac{1}{2}.(0.912+0.707) \\ &= 0.809 \end{aligned}$$

AUC may also be calculated from the maximal Youden index at this threshold, which is 0.619 (Sect. 4.2):

$$\begin{aligned} AUC &= \tfrac{1}{2}.(Y+1) \\ &= \tfrac{1}{2}.(0.619+1) \\ &= 0.809 \end{aligned}$$

Hence, treating MACE as a binary classifier with a single fixed threshold underestimates AUC compared to the full ROC plot (= 0.886) [41].

AUC may also be calculated from DOR = 25.06 at this MACE cut-off:

$$\begin{aligned} AUC &= DOR/(DOR-1)^2.\left[(DOR-1)-\log_e(DOR)\right] \\ &= 0.0433\times 20.839 \\ &= 0.902 \end{aligned}$$

This is greater than the AUC value calculated from Sens and Spec (0.809), presumably because the equation assumes the ROC curve to be symmetric with DOR = 25.06.

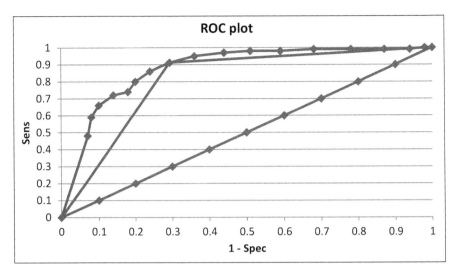

**Fig. 6.3** ROC plot for MACE for the diagnosis of dementia versus no dementia, comparing MACE as a continuous scale (upper curve, = same as Fig. 6.1) or as a single fixed threshold binary classifier (lower triangle), with chance diagonal (y = x) [41]

## 6.2.1   Defining Optimal Cut-Off: Youden Index (Y)

As previously discussed (Sect. 4.2), Youden index (Y) is a global or unitary measure of test performance given by Y = Sens + Spec − 1.

The maximal value of Y corresponds to the point on the ROC curve which is the maximal vertical distance from the diagonal line (y = x) which represents the performance of a random classifier. Also known as c*, this point minimizes misclassification (the sum of FPR and FNR) [52]:

$$
\begin{aligned}
Y_{\backprime} &= \max\left[\operatorname{Sens}(c*) + \operatorname{Spec}(c*) - 1\right] \\
&= \max \operatorname{Sens}(c*) - \operatorname{FPR}(c*) \\
&= \min\left[\left(\operatorname{FPR}(c*) + \operatorname{FNR}(c*)\right)\right]
\end{aligned}
$$

In error notation:

$$
\begin{aligned}
Y &= \max\left[(1-\beta) + (1-\alpha) - 1\right] \\
&= \min\left[(\alpha + \beta)\right]
\end{aligned}
$$

The cut-point maximising Sens and Spec is the point on the ROC curve which also represents the minimization of expected costs if and only if the cost of FN

**Table 6.2** MACE sensitivity, specificity, and predictive values at optimal cut-off values as defined by various global parameters (Data from [28, 30, 31, 33, 35])

| Optimal cut-off | Metric used to define optimal cut-off | Sens | Spec | Y | PPV | NPV | PSI |
|---|---|---|---|---|---|---|---|
| ≤13/30 | LDM (= NNM/NNP) | 0.48 | 0.93 | 0.41 | 0.57 | 0.91 | 0.48 |
| ≤14/30 | Acc<br>LDM (= NNM/NNP) | 0.59 | 0.92 | 0.51 | 0.56 | 0.93 | 0.49 |
| ≤15/30 | CSI<br>F measure<br>HMYPSI<br>MCC<br>LDM (= NNM/NND)<br>SUI | 0.66 | 0.90 | 0.56 | 0.53 | 0.94 | 0.47 |
| ≤18/30 | Q* index (graphically) | 0.80 | 0.80 | 0.60 | 0.42 | 0.96 | 0.38 |
| ≤19/30 | Euclidean index (d) | 0.86 | 0.76 | 0.62 | 0.38 | 0.97 | 0.35 |
| ≤20/30 | Youden index (Y) | 0.91 | 0.71 | 0.62 | 0.36 | 0.98 | 0.34 |
| ≤23/30 | DOR<br>Q* index (calculated) | 0.98 | 0.49 | 0.47 | 0.25 | 0.99 | 0.24 |

Abbreviations: *Acc* correct classification accuracy, *CSI* critical success index, *DOR* diagnostic odds ratio, *HMYPSI* harmonic mean of Y and PSI, *LDM* likelihood to be diagnosed or misdiagnosed, *MCC* Matthews' correlation coefficient, *NND* number needed to diagnose, *NNM* number needed to misdiagnose, *NNP* number needed to predict, *NPV* negative predictive index, *PPV* positive predictive index, *PSI* predictive summary index, *Sens* sensitivity, *Spec* specificity, *SUI* summary utility index, *Y* Youden index

(misclassifying the diseased as undiseased) is equal to the cost of FP (misclassifying the undiseased as diseased) [22]. As previously discussed, this equivalence rarely if ever holds in clinical practice (Sect. 3.2.5).

In a study examining the Mini-Addenbrooke's Cognitive Examination (MACE) [18], optimal cut-off defined using the maximal Youden index was ≤20/30. This cut-off gave a relatively good balance of test sensitivity and specificity (Table 6.2) [28, 31].

## 6.2.2   Defining Optimal Cut-Off: Euclidean Index (d)

The Euclidean index (d) is the point minimally distant from the top left hand ("north west") corner of the ROC plot, with coordinates (0,1), with the ROC intersect of a line joining these points designated c [6, 60], such that:

$$
\begin{aligned}
d &= \min \sqrt{\left[\left(1-\mathrm{Sens}(c)\right)^2 + \left(1-\mathrm{Spec}(c)\right)^2\right]} \\
&= \min \sqrt{\left[\left(\mathrm{FNR}(c)\right)^2 + \left(\mathrm{FPR}(c)\right)^2\right]}
\end{aligned}
$$

Hence this will be seen to minimize the misclassification rate (Sect. 3.2.5). When c and c* (Sect. 7.2.1) do not agree, c* is deemed preferable since it maximizes the overall rate of correct classification ([58], p. 51–2).

In a study examining the MACE, optimal cut-off defined using the minimal Euclidean index was ≤19/30, giving a relatively good balance of sensitivity and specificity (Table 6.2) [31].

### 6.2.3  Defining Optimal Cut-Off: Q* Index

Using a summary ROC (SROC) curve based on data from meta-analyses, another index was proposed to determine optimal test cut-off: the Q* index. This is the point where the downward, negative, or anti-diagonal line through unit ROC space (y = 1 − x, or Sens = Spec, or Sens − Spec = 0, or TPR = 1 − FPR) intersects the ROC curve [43] (Fig. 6.4). Q* index may also be defined as the "point of indifference on the ROC curve", where the sensitivity and specificity are equal, or, in other words, where the probabilities of incorrect test results are equal for disease cases and non-cases (i.e. indifference between false positive and false negative diagnostic errors, with both assumed to be of equal value). For the particular case of a symmetrical ROC curve, Q* will be equal to the Euclidean index [54].

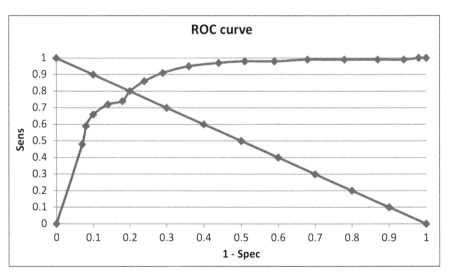

**Fig. 6.4**  ROC curve for diagnosis of dementia using MACE (= same as Fig. 6.1), intersecting with the anti-diagonal (y = 1 − x) line for assessment of Q* index. (Modified from [28])

**Worked Example: Q\* Index**

A ROC plot of the results of the MACE study [28] intersected with the anti-diagonal line $(y = 1 - x)$ through unit ROC space, the Q\* index, at 0.8 (Fig. 6.4), corresponding to an optimal MACE cut-off value of $\leq 18/30$, where Sens = Spec = 0.8.

Q\* index was also calculated from DOR. The MACE ROC plot is not symmetric, so DOR varies with test cut-off, with a maximal value of 52.8 at MACE cut-off of $\leq 23/30$ [31].

Hence the value for Q\* index [54] using this DOR was:

$$
\begin{aligned}
Q^* &= \sqrt{DOR} / \left[ 1 + \sqrt{DOR} \right] \\
&= \sqrt{52.8} / \left[ 1 + \sqrt{52.8} \right] \\
&= 0.879
\end{aligned}
$$

At this cut-off, Sens = 0.98 and Spec = 0.49, a poorer balance than seen with the graphical estimation of Q\* index (Table 6.2) [30].

Q\* index has also been suggested as useful global measure of test accuracy [26], although its use for the comparison of diagnostic tests is controversial and has been generally discouraged [36].

As well as being assessed graphically, as the point of intersection of the ROC curve and the anti-diagonal through ROC space (Fig. 6.4), Q\* index may also be calculated based on its relationship to the diagnostic odds ratio (DOR; Sect. 2.4.1). Q\* may be calculated [54] as:

$$
Q^* = \sqrt{DOR} / \left[ 1 + \sqrt{DOR} \right]
$$

### 6.2.4   Defining Optimal Cut-Off: Other ROC-Based Methods

Other ROC-based methods to define optimal cut-off are described. In the "empirical method" [37], also known as the "product index" [14], a concordance probability maximizing the product of Sens and Spec is used. Another method uses the maximal "number needed to misdiagnose" [12] (Sect. 5.4) weighted according to an estimate of the relative costs of FN and FP test results [13].

### 6.2.5   Defining Optimal Cut-Off: Diagnostic Odds Ratio (DOR)

Maximal diagnostic odds ratio (DOR; Sect. 2.4.1) or its logarithm has frequently been used to define test cut-points. However, some authors have recommended against use of DOR because it produces a concave curve, and hence extremely high and low cut-points [2, 14]. Examining the MACE study data [31], maximal DOR cut-off (≤23/30) was an outlier compared to other ROC and non-ROC methods (as for Q* index calculated from DOR; Sect. 6.2.3 [30]), resulting in a high sensitivity but poor specificity test performance (Table 6.2).

### 6.2.6   Defining Optimal Cut-Off: Non-ROC-Based Methods

Various other global or unitary measures may be used to define test cut-off [31], for example maximal accuracy (Sect. 3.2.4) or kappa (Sect. 7.2.2), critical success index (Sect. 4.8) [35], F measure (Sect. 4.9), Matthews' correlation coefficient (Sect. 4.5), summary utility index (Sect. 4.10) [33] and the two formulations of the likelihood to be diagnosed of misdiagnosed (LDM and LPM; Sect. 5.5) [33].

In the study examining MACE, optimal cut-offs defined by these measures clustered around ≤13/30 to ≤15/30, resulting in greater specificity than sensitivity (Table 6.2) [31, 35].

## 6.3   Other Graphing Methods

A number of other graphing methods which display some of the measures derived from a 2 × 2 contingency table have been reported. None has achieved the breadth of usage of the ROC plot.

### 6.3.1   ROC Plot in Likelihood Ratio Coordinates

Johnson advocated transformation of ROC curves into positive and negative likelihood ratio (LR+, LR−; Sect. 2.3.4) coordinates, in part because half the potential region for ROC curves was deemed to have no meaning [20] (test performance falling in the area below the diagonal is an outcome worse than random guessing; this has been termed the "perverse zone" [48]).

Using logarithmic scales, optimal LR ROC curves bend further from the lower left corner, where $\log_{10}LR+ = \log_{10}LR- = 0$, and towards the upper right ("north east") area where $\log_{10}LR+$ and $\log_{10}LR-$ approach infinity. The slope of the LR ROC curve equals the log diagnostic odds ratio at that point (whereas the slope of

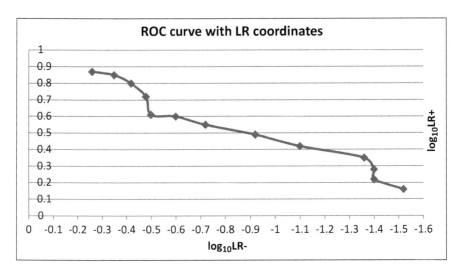

**Fig. 6.5** ROC curve with LR coordinates for diagnosis of dementia using MACE. (Data from [28])

**Fig. 6.6** Precision-recall (PR) plot or curve for diagnosis of dementia using MACE. (Modified from [28])

the ROC curve in its usual coordinates of Sens and 1 – Spec equals LR; Sect. 6.2). Using the transformed axes, AUC = 0 is a useless test, rather than 0.5 in the usual ROC plot. Comparison of tests is also possible using this method, as for regret graphs [17].

An attempt to convert data from the MACE study [28] to likelihood ratio coordinates is shown in Fig. 6.5 (compare with the conventional ROC plot of Fig. 6.1).

### 6.3.2  Precision-Recall (PR) Plot or Curve

The precision recall (PR) plot or curve is, like the ROC plot, a performance graphing method. It plots precision or positive predictive value (Sect. 2.3.1) on the ordinate against recall or sensitivity (Sect. 2.2.1) on the abscissa with linear interpolation between points [8] (Fig. 6.6). Like ROC curves, PR curves may be described as "threshold free".

PR curves avoid some of the "optimism" of ROC curves [7, 45] and are more informative than ROC curves when analysing skewed datasets [50]. Area under the PR curve may be calculated, although this is not straightforward [23], and visual interpretation may be adequate to denote better classification performance (as for ROC curves). Little use has been made of PR curves in assessing clinical diagnostic and screening tests [28].

### 6.3.3  Prevalence Value Accuracy Plots

Prevalence value accuracy contour plots attempt to include the cost of misclassifications (FP and FN; z-axis) as well as prevalence (x-axis) and unit cost ratio (y-axis) in graphing test performance. A derived misclassification index may give a different interpretation of the relative merit of tests compared to AUC ROC [47].

### 6.3.4  Agreement Charts

The agreement chart is a two-dimensional graph permitting visual assessment of the agreement or concordance between two observers. Unlike the kappa statistic (Sect. 7.2.2), the agreement chart helps to uncover patterns of disagreement between observers, but it can only be used for ordinal scale variables [1].

## 6.4  Effect Sizes

There are many effect size measures, which may be broadly categorised into: measures of association (the $r$ family), of which the phi ($\varphi$) coefficient (as Matthews' correlation coefficient) has already been described (Sect. 4.5); and differences between groups (the $d$ family) [10]. The latter group, specifically Cohen's $d$, is the focus of this section.

Fig. 6.7  Cohen's *d*
formula

Cohen's *d* formula:

$$d = \frac{\overline{X}_1 - \overline{X}_2}{\sqrt{\dfrac{s_1^2 + s_2^2}{2}}}$$

Where *d* = Cohen's *d* effect size
$X_1$ and $X_2$ = means of two groups
$s_1$ and $s_2$ = standard deviations of two groups

**Table 6.3**  Classification of Cohen's *d* (After [4, 5, 50])

|           | Huge   | Very large | Large  | Medium | Small  | Very poor |
|-----------|--------|------------|--------|--------|--------|-----------|
| Cohen's *d* | ≥ 2.00 | ≥ 1.20     | ≥ 0.80 | ≥ 0.50 | ≥ 0.20 | ≥ 0.01    |

## 6.4.1  Correlation Coefficient

Correlation coefficients, of which the best known is Pearson's product moment correlation coefficient (*r*), quantify the strength of relationship between two variables which may be either dichotomous or continuous. Correlations vary between +1 (perfect positive linear relationship) through 0 (no relationship between variables) to −1 (perfect negative linear relationship).

## 6.4.2  Cohen's d

Cohen's *d* effect size [4] is calculated as the difference of the means of the two groups being compared divided by the weighted pooled standard deviations of the groups (Fig. 6.7) if they are roughly the same (if not, then other options such as Glass's Δ or Hedges' *g* may be more appropriate [10]). Rules of thumb for the qualitative classification of Cohen's *d* effect size were given by Cohen [4, 5] and updated by Sawilowsky [51] (Table 6.3).

Hence Cohen's *d* is not calculated on the basis of the 2 × 2 contingency table; it is independent of cut point, and of base rate. Nevertheless, like AUC ROC (Sect. 6.2), Cohen's *d* quantifies the amount of separation between the distribution of scores for groups with and without the criterion diagnosis ([57], p. 208). Cohen's *d* may be used to compare between tests, such as cognitive screening instruments [25, 27], and values may change with disease prevalence [56].

As both Cohen's *d* and *r* are standardised, they can be interconverted [10], e.g.

$$r = d / \sqrt{d^2 + 4}$$

**Worked Examples: Cohen's d**
In a large (N = 755) screening test accuracy study of MACE [28], a reference (criterion) diagnosis of dementia, based on the application of widely accepted diagnostic criteria for dementia, was made in 114 patients; the remaining patients without dementia (n = 641) had either mild cognitive impairment (MCI; n = 222) or subjective memory complaints (SMC; n = 419).

In the dementia group, mean MACE test score +/− standard deviation was 13.56 +/− 5.19. In the non-demented group, the mean score was 22.39 +/− 4.98. Hence;

$$d = 22.39 - 13.56 / \sqrt{\left(5.19^2 + 4.98^2 / 2\right)}$$
$$= 8.83 / 5.09$$
$$= 1.74$$

According to the suggested classification of Cohen's $d$ values (Table 6.3), this was a very large effect size.

Comparing MACE scores in the MCI group (mean = 19.09 +/− 4.78) with the SMC group (24.14 +/− 4.12):

$$d = 24.14 - 19.09 / \sqrt{\left(4.78^2 + 4.12^2 / 2\right)}$$
$$= 5.05 / 4.46$$
$$= 1.13$$

According to the classification (Table 6.3), this was a large effect size [28].

To examine the change in various metrics with disease prevalence, values were calculated for those aged ≥65 (n = 287) and ≥75 years (n = 119) comparing the dementia group with the non-dementia group [34]. In the ≥65 years group the mean MACE score in the dementia group was = 13.65 +/− 4.93 and in the non-dementia group it was 21.81 +/− 4.77. Hence calculating for Cohen's $d$:

$$d = 21.81 - 13.65 / \sqrt{\left(4.93^2 + 4.77^2 / 2\right)}$$
$$= 8.16 / 4.85$$
$$= 1.68$$

According to the classification (Table 6.3), this was a very large effect size.

For the ≥75 years group, mean MACE score in the dementia group was = 13.07 +/− 4.62 and in the non-dementia group was 19.58 +/− 4.37:

$$d = 19.58 - 13.07 / \sqrt{\left(4.62^2 + 4.37^2 / 2\right)}$$
$$= 6.51 / 4.50$$
$$= 1.45$$

According to the classification (Table 6.3), this was a very large effect size (Larner, unpublished observations).

## 6.4.3 Binomial Effect Size Display (BESD)

The binomial effect size display (BESD) is a 2 × 2 contingency table designed to present correlational effects in a manner indicating the "real-world" importance of the findings [49].

Correlation is expressed as a success rate difference, in rows expressing independent variables (e.g. treatment and control groups) and columns expressing any dependent variable which can be dichotomised (e.g. success, failure). For a given correlation, $r$, success rate is calculated for treatment and control groups as $0.5 +/- r/2$, each column and row summing to 100. However it has been argued that success rate differences may be biased by various factors and overestimate these values [19, 46].

---

**Worked Example: Binomial Effect Size Display (BESD)**
In the screening test accuracy study of MACE [28], it was found that for the diagnosis of dementia Cohen's $d$ effect size = 1.74. To display this finding in a "real-world" manner, a binomial effect size display (BESD) was constructed. Firstly, $r$ was calculated from Cohen's $d$:

$$r = d / \sqrt{d^2 + 4}$$
$$= 1.74 / \sqrt{1.74^2 + 4}$$
$$= 0.656$$

For this correlation, success rate was calculated for patients diagnosed with and without dementia as $0.5 +/- r/2 = 0.172$ and $0.828$. Hence, the BESD:

| | Criterion diagnosis: dementia | Criterion diagnosis: no dementia |
|---|---|---|
| MACE diagnosis: dementia | 82.8 | 17.2 |
| MACE diagnosis: no dementia | 17.2 | 82.8 |

Diagnosis was therefore about five times more successful than unsuccessful. This gives a more optimistic result than the likelihood to be diagnosed or misdiagnosed (LDM) metric (Sect. 5.5): even at the optimal MACE cut-off defined by maximal LDM = NNM/NND, ≤15/30 (Table 6.2), the unrounded LDM was only 3.94.

# References

1. Bangdiwala SI, Shankar V. The agreement chart. BMC Med Res Methodol. 2013;13:97.
2. Bohning D, Holling H, Patilea V. A limitation of the diagnostic-odds ratio in determining an optimal cut-off value for a continuous diagnostic test. Stat Methods Med Res. 2011;20:541–50.
3. Choi BC. Slopes of a receiver operating characteristic curve and likelihood ratios for a diagnostic test. Am J Epidemiol. 1998;148:1127–32.
4. Cohen J. Statistical power analysis for the behavioral sciences. 2nd ed. Hillsdale: Lawrence Erlbaum; 1988.
5. Cohen J. A power primer. Psychol Bull. 1992;112:155–9.
6. Coffin M, Sukhatme S. Receiver operating characteristic studies and measurement errors. Biometrics. 1997;53:823–37.
7. Cook J, Ramadas V. When to consult precision-recall curves. Stata J. 2020;20:131–48.
8. Davis J, Goadrich M. The relationship between Precision-Recall and ROC curves. In: ICML '06: Proceedings of the 23rd International Conference on Machine Learning. New York: ACM; 2006, p. 233–40.
9. DeLong ER, DeLong DM, Clarke-Pearson DL. Comparing the areas under two or more correlated receiver operating characteristic curves: a nonparametric approach. Biometrics. 1988;44:837–45.
10. Ellis PD. The essential guide to effect sizes: statistical power, meta-analysis, and the interpretation of research results. Cambridge: Cambridge University Press; 2010.
11. Fawcett T. An introduction to ROC analysis. Pattern Recogn Lett. 2006;27:861–74.
12. Habibzadeh F, Yadollahie M. Number needed to misdiagnose: a measure of diagnostic test effectiveness. Epidemiology. 2013;24:170.
13. Habibzadeh F, Habibzadeh P, Yadollahie M. On determining the most appropriate test cut-off value: the case of tests with continuous results. Biochem Med (Zagreb). 2016;26:297–307.
14. Hajian-Tilaki K. The choice of methods in determining the optimal cut-off value for quantitative diagnostic test evaluation. Stat Methods Med Res. 2018;27:2374–83.
15. Hanley JA, McNeil BJ. The meaning and use of the area under a receiver operating characteristic (ROC) curve. Radiology. 1982;143:29–36.
16. Hanley JA, McNeil BJ. A method of comparing the areas under receiver operating characteristic curves derived from the same cases. Radiology. 1983;148:839–43.
17. Hilden J, Glasziou P. Regret graphs, diagnostic uncertainty and Youden's index. Stat Med. 1996;15:969–86.
18. Hsieh S, McGrory S, Leslie F, Dawson K, Ahmed S, Butler CR, et al. The Mini-Addenbrooke's Cognitive Examination: a new assessment tool for dementia. Dement Geriatr Cogn Disord. 2015;39:1–11.
19. Hsu LM. Biases of success rate differences shown in binomial effect size displays. Psychol Methods. 2004;9:183–97.
20. Johnson NP. Advantages to transforming the receiver operating characteristic (ROC) curve into likelihood ratio co-ordinates. Stat Med. 2004;23:2257–66.
21. Jones CM, Athanasiou T. Summary receiver operating characteristic curve analysis techniques in the evaluation of diagnostic tests. Ann Thorac Surg. 2005;79:16–20.
22. Kaivanto K. Maximization of the sum of sensitivity and specificity as a diagnostic cutpoint criterion. J Clin Epidemiol. 2008;61:516–7.
23. Keilwagen J, Grosse I, Grau J. Area under precision-recall curves for weighted and unweighted data. PLoS One. 2014;9(3):e92209.
24. Krzanowski WJ, Hand DJ. ROC curves for continuous data. New York: CRC Press; 2009.
25. Larner AJ. Effect size (Cohen's d) of cognitive screening instruments examined in pragmatic diagnostic accuracy studies. Dement Geriatr Cogn Disord Extra. 2014;4:236–41.
26. Larner AJ. The Q* index: a useful global measure of dementia screening test accuracy? Dement Geriatr Cogn Dis Extra. 2015;5:265–70.

27. Larner AJ. Cognitive screening instruments for the diagnosis of mild cognitive impairment. Prog Neurol Psychiatry. 2016;20(2):21–6.
28. Larner AJ. MACE for diagnosis of dementia and MCI: examining cut-offs and predictive values. Diagnostics (Basel). 2019;9:E51.
29. Larner AJ. What is test accuracy? Comparing unitary accuracy metrics for cognitive screening instruments. Neurodegener Dis Manag. 2019;9:277–81.
30. Larner AJ. Screening for dementia: Q* index as a global measure of test accuracy revisited. medRxiv. 2020. https://doi.org/10.1101/2020.04.01.20050567.
31. Larner AJ. Defining "optimal" test cut-off using global test metrics: evidence from a cognitive screening instrument. Neurodegener Dis Manag. 2020;10:223–30.
32. Larner AJ. The "attended alone" and "attended with" signs in the assessment of cognitive impairment: a revalidation. Postgrad Med. 2020;132:595–600.
33. Larner AJ. Manual of screeners for dementia: pragmatic test accuracy studies. London: Springer; 2020.
34. Larner AJ. Mini-Addenbrooke's Cognitive Examination (MACE): a useful cognitive screening instrument in older people? Can Geriatr J. 2020;23:199–204.
35. Larner AJ. Assessing cognitive screening instruments with the critical success index. Prog Neurol Psychiatry. 2021;25(3):33–7.
36. Lee J, Kim KW, Choi SH, Huh J, Park SH. Systematic review and meta-analysis of studies evaluating diagnostic test accuracy: a practical review for clinical researchers – part II. Statistical methods of meta-analysis. Korean J Radiol. 2015;16:1188–96.
37. Liu X. Classification accuracy and cut point selection. Stat Med. 2012;31:2676–86.
38. Lusted L. Introduction to medical decision making. Springfield: Charles Thomas; 1968.
39. Lusted LB. Signal detectability and medical decision-making. Science. 1971;171:1217–9.
40. Mallett S, Halligan S, Thompson M, Collins GS, Altman DG. Interpreting diagnostic accuracy studies for patient care. BMJ. 2012;345:e3999.
41. Mbizvo GK, Larner AJ. Receiver operating characteristic plot and area under the curve with binary classifiers: pragmatic analysis of cognitive screening instruments. Neurodegener Dis Manag. 2021;11:353–60.
42. Metz CE. Basic principles of ROC analysis. Semin Nucl Med. 1978;8:283–98.
43. Moses LE, Shapiro D, Littenberg B. Combining independent studies of a diagnostic test into a summary ROC curve: data-analytic approaches and some additional considerations. Stat Med. 1993;12:1293–316.
44. Muschelli J. ROC and AUC with a binary predictor: a potentially misleading metric. J Classif. 2020;37:696–708.
45. Ozenne B, Subtil F, Maucort-Boulch D. The precision-recall curve overcame the optimism of the receiver operating characteristic curve in rare diseases. J Clin Epidemiol. 2015;68:855–9.
46. Randolph JJ, Edmondson RS. Using the binomial effect size display to present the magnitude of effect sizes to the evaluation audience. Pract Assess Res Eval. 2005;10:14.
47. Remaley AT, Sampson ML, DeLeo JM, Remaley NA, Farsi BD, Zweig MH. Prevalence-value-accuracy plots: a new method for comparing diagnostic tests based on misclassification costs. Clin Chem. 1999;45:934–41.
48. Richardson ML. The zombie plot: a simple graphic method for visualizing the efficacy of a diagnostic test. AJR Am J Roentgenol. 2016;207:W43–52.
49. Rosenthal R, Rubin DR. A simple, general purpose display of magnitude of experimental effect. J Educ Psychol. 1982;74:166–9.
50. Saito T, Rehmsmeier M. The precision-recall plot is more informative than the ROC plot when evaluating binary classifiers on imbalanced datasets. PLoS One. 2015;10(3):e0118432.
51. Sawilowsky SS. New effect sizes rules of thumb. J Mod Appl Stat Methods. 2009;8:597–9.
52. Schisterman EF, Perkins NJ, Liu A, Bondell H. Optimal cut-point and its corresponding Youden Index to discriminate individuals using pooled blood samples. Epidemiology. 2005;16:73–81.
53. Swets JA. Measuring the accuracy of diagnostic systems. Science. 1988;240:1285–93.

54. Walter SD. Properties of the summary receiver operating characteristic (SROC) curve for diagnostic test data. Stat Med. 2002;21:1237–56.

55. Weiskrantz L. Blindsight. A case study and implications, Oxford Psychology Series No. 12. Oxford: Clarendon Press; 1986.

56. Wojtowicz A, Larner AJ. Diagnostic test accuracy of cognitive screeners in older people. Prog Neurol Psychiatry. 2017;21(1):17–21.

57. Youngstrom EA. A primer on receiver operating characteristic analysis and diagnostic efficiency statistics for pediatric psychology: we are ready to ROC. J Pediatr Psychol. 2014;39:204–21.

58. Zhou XH, Obuchowski NA, McClish DK. Statistical methods in diagnostic medicine. 2nd ed. Hoboken: Wiley; 2011.

59. Zou KH, O'Malley J, Mauri L. Receiver-operating characteristic analysis for evaluating diagnostic tests and predictive models. Circulation. 2007;115:654–7.

60. Zweig MH, Campbell G. Receiver-operating characteristic (ROC) plots: a fundamental evaluation tool in clinical medicine. Clin Chem. 1993;39:561–77.

# Chapter 7
# Other Measures, Other Tables

## Contents

## 7.1 Introduction

$2 \times 2$ contingency tables may be used for purposes other than generating the various measures which have been discussed in Chaps. 2, 3, 4, 5, and 6. There are methods, based on the $2 \times 2$ contingency table, to assess association and agreement between measures. Other measures of association, such as correlation coefficient, have already been described (Sect. 6.3.1).

## 7.2 Other measures

### 7.2.1 Measure of Association: McNemar's Test

The test first described by McNemar [45] examines paired nominal data in a $2 \times 2$ contingency table to determine whether row and column marginal frequencies are equal. It tests the null hypothesis of marginal homogeneity.

© Springer Nature Switzerland AG 2021
A. J. Larner, *The 2x2 Matrix*, https://doi.org/10.1007/978-3-030-74920-0_7

In algebraic notation (see Fig. 1.2):

$$\chi^2 = (b-c)^2 / (b+c)$$

This may sometimes be expressed by representing the larger number of pairs as $n_1$ and the smaller as $n_2$:

$$\chi^2 = (n_1 - n_2)^2 / (n_1 + n_2)$$

When numbers are small $(b + c < 25)$, a continuity correction is applied [19]:

$$\chi^2 = [(b-c)-1]^2 / (b+c)$$

or:

$$\chi^2 = [(n_1 - n_2)-1]^2 / (n_1 + n_2)$$

**Worked Examples: McNemar Test of Association**
In a study examining memory complaints in patients attending a dedicated epilepsy clinic $(N = 100)$ [2], easily dichotomised screeners for both mood [4] and sleep disturbance [27, 29] were administered. There was a statistically significant difference in sleep disturbance and mood disturbance between the patients who reported subjective memory complaints and those who did not.

McNemar's test of association was used to examine whether there was a statistically significant association between disturbed sleep and disturbed mood in this patient cohort. Twenty patients had disturbed mood but not disturbed sleep (b), whereas 6 patients had disturbed sleep but not disturbed mood (c). Hence:

$$\begin{aligned}
\chi^2 &= (b-c)^2 / (b+c) \\
&= (20-6)^2 / (20+6) \\
&= 196 / 26 \\
&= 7.538 \\
p &= 0.009
\end{aligned}$$

Hence a statistically significant association between disturbed sleep and disturbed mood was found in this cohort of epilepsy patients, permitting rejection of the null hypothesis [2].

McNemar's test of association was used similarly in a study of patients diagnosed with functional cognitive disorders $(N = 44)$ [6] to examine whether there was a statistically significant association between disturbed sleep and disturbed mood, using the same screeners for these constructs [4, 27, 29]. Five patients had disturbed mood but not disturbed sleep (b), whereas 6 patients had disturbed sleep but not disturbed mood (c). Hence, since b + c < 25, a continuity correction [19] was applied:

$$\chi^2 = \left[(b-c)-1\right]^2 / (b+c)$$

or, since c > b:

$$\chi^2 = \left[(n_1 - n_2)-1\right]^2 / (n_1 + n_2)$$

Let $n_1 = 6$, $n_2 = 5$:

$$\chi^2 = \left[(6-5)-1\right]^2 / (6+5)$$
$$= 0/11$$
$$= 0$$
$$p = 1$$

Hence no statistically significant association between disturbed sleep and disturbed mood was found in this patient cohort [39].

Using data from the same study [6], the association between mood [4] and subjective memory complaint assessed with a dichotomised Likert scale [49] was also examined (N = 44). Four patients had disturbed mood but not subjective memory complaint (b), whereas 8 patients had subjective memory complaint but not disturbed mood (c). Again, a continuity correction was applied, since b + c < 25. As c > b, let $n_1 = 8$, $n_2 = 4$:

$$\chi^2 = \left[(n_1 - n_2)-1\right]^2 / (n_1 + n_2)$$
$$= \left[(8-4)-1\right]^2 / (8+4)$$
$$= 9/12$$
$$= 0.75$$
$$p = 0.39$$

Hence no statistically significant association between subjective memory complaint and disturbed mood was found in this patient cohort [39].

**Worked Example: McNemar Test of Association**
Two brief cognitive screening instruments, the Mini-Cog [8] and the cognitive disorders examination (Codex) [5], were examined in a screening test accuracy study (N = 162) [40]. Using test cut-offs for dementia from the index studies, 16 patients categorised as "not dementia" by Codex were categorized as "dementia" by Mini-Cog, whereas in only 3 patients was the reverse discordance observed. Hence, since b + c < 25, a continuity correction [19] was applied:

$$\chi^2 = \left[(b-c)-1\right]^2/(b+c)$$
$$= \left[(16-3)-1\right]^2/(16+3)$$
$$= 144/19$$
$$= 7.579$$
$$p = 0.0059$$

Hence the null hypothesis of marginal homogeneity was rejected. The marginal proportions were significantly different from each other. This is probably related to the better specificity of Codex than Mini-Cog for dementia diagnosis (Larner, unpublished observations).

As will be noted, McNemar's test is a test of the null hypothesis, with resultant conditional probability $p$ values. The shortcomings of $p$ values are well-recognised (Sect. 1.5), as they confound effect size with sample size, and a value "dichotomised" as significant at $p < 0.05$ is not a guarantee that a result is real (it could still be a false positive result or type I error), nor that a value deemed non-significant at $p > 0.05$ is inconclusive (it could still be a false negative result or type II error). The practice of using $p$ values is increasingly controversial, with some advocating their "retirement" [3].

## 7.2.2 Measure of Agreement: Cohen's Kappa (κ) Statistic

The kappa statistic, κ, is usually designated as a measure of agreement or concordance beyond chance, for example between different observers, assessors or raters, or between different screening or diagnostic tests [15]. This is calculated by comparing the proportion of observed agreement, $P_a$, with the proportion of agreement expected by chance alone, $P_c$, for a total of N observations, where:

$$\kappa = \left(P_a - P_c\right)/\left(1 - P_c\right)$$

In algebraic notation (see Fig. 1.2):

$$P_a = (a+d)/N$$

Note that this corresponds to the definition previously given for Accuracy (Acc; Sect. 3.2.4). Hence this may also be expressed as:

$$\kappa = (Acc - P_c)/(1 - P_c)$$

The proportion of agreement expected by chance alone, $P_c$, is given by:

$$P_c = (a+b)(a+c)/N^2 + (c+d)(b+d)/N^2$$

Hence:

$$\kappa = (a+d)/N - \left[(a+b)(a+c)/N^2 + (c+d)(b+d)/N^2\right]/$$
$$1 - (a+b)(a+c)/N^2 + (c+d)(b+d)/N^2$$

or:

$$\kappa = 2(ad - bc)/\left[(a+c)(c+d) + (a+b)(b+d)\right]$$

$\kappa$ ranges from +1 to −1, with most values expected to fall within the range 0 (agreement due to chance alone) to 1 (perfect agreement), with negative values occurring only when agreement occurs less often than predicted by chance alone, a rare situation in clinical practice. Interpretation of $\kappa$ values is often based on the convention of Landis and Koch [30]: very good agreement (>0.8–1.0), good agreement (>0.6–0.8), moderate agreement (>0.4–0.6), fair agreement (>0.2–0.4), slight agreement (0–0.2), and poor agreement worse than chance (<0).

**Worked Example: Accuracy with Kappa Statistic**
The Mini-Addenbrooke's Cognitive Examination (MACE) [25] was examined in a large (N = 755) prospective screening test accuracy study [35]. At the MACE cut-off of ≤20/30 the test outcomes were as follows: a (=TP) = 104, b (=FP) = 188, c (=FN) = 10, and d (=TN) = 453 (Fig. 2.2). Hence:

$$P_a = (a+d)/N$$
$$= 557/755$$
$$= 0.738$$
$$= Acc \ (see \ Sect. \ 3.2.4)$$

$$P_c = (a+b)(a+c)/N^2 + (c+d)(b+d)/N^2$$
$$= 292 \times 114 / 755^2 + 463 \times 641 / 755^2$$
$$= 33288/570025 + 296783/570025$$
$$= 0.0584 + 0.521$$
$$= 0.579$$

$$\kappa = (P_a - P_c)/(1-P_c)$$
$$= (0.738 - 0.579)/(1 - 0.579)$$
$$= 0.159/0.421$$
$$= 0.378$$

Note that this result agrees with the calculation of "unbiased Acc" (= 0.378) shown in Sect. 3.2.4.

This may also be calculated using:

$$\kappa = 2(ad-bc)/\left[(a+c)(c+d)+(a+b)(b+d)\right]$$
$$= 2 \times 45232 / \left[(114 \times 463)+(292 \times 641)\right]$$
$$= 2 \times 45232 / 52782 + 187172$$
$$= 90464/239954$$
$$= 0.377$$

[The different results relate to rounding errors.]

De Vet et al. [18] argued that Cohen's kappa is a relative measure, adjusting observed agreement for expected agreement, and hence is in fact a measure of reliability rather than a measure of agreement, hence accounting for the observation of instances of high agreement with low kappa and vice versa, for example in cases of class imbalance. Bangdiwala's B statistic is another summary measure of concordance.

Despite these caveats, Cohen's kappa may also be used for the comparison of assessors and the comparison of tests, as demonstrated in the following examples.

**Worked Example: Cohen's Kappa ($\kappa$) Statistic – Comparison of Assessors**

The Ascertain Dementia 8 (AD8) cognitive screening questionnaire was used in a study examining the frequency of cognitive impairment in patients with epilepsy [1]. AD8 may be administered to both patients [24] and informants [23]. The AD8 cut-off from the index studies was used, where a score $\geq 2/8$ indicates cognitive impairment is likely to be present.

In the study population (N = 100), there were 44 patient:informant dyads for whom both self-rated and informant AD8 scores were available. 21/44 patients self-rated AD8 $\geq 2/8$, and 24/44 informants rated patients' AD8 score $\geq 2/8$, with agreement in 21 dyads. 23/44 patients self-rated AD8 $<2/8$ and 20/44 informants rated patients' AD8 score $<2/8$, with agreement in 20 dyads. Constructing a $2 \times 2$ table the values for a, b, c, and d were therefore 21, 3, 0, and 20 respectively,

Hence observed agreement was:

$$
\begin{aligned}
P_a &= (a+d)/N \\
&= (21+20)/44 \\
&= 0.932
\end{aligned}
$$

Agreement expected by chance was:

$$
\begin{aligned}
P_c &= (a+b)(a+c)/N^2 + (c+d)(b+d)/N^2 \\
&= (21+3)(21+0)/44^2 + (0+20)(3+20)/44^2 \\
&= 0.260 + 0.238 \\
&= 0.498
\end{aligned}
$$

Therefore:

$$
\begin{aligned}
\kappa &= (P_a - P_c)/(1-P_c) \\
&= (0.932-0.498)/(1-0.498) \\
&= 0.864
\end{aligned}
$$

Based on the convention of Landis and Koch [30], this value of $\kappa$ would be interpreted as very good agreement ($>0.8$–$1.0$).

**Worked Example: Cohen's Kappa (κ) Statistic – Comparison of Screening Tests**

Two cognitive screening instruments, the Mini-Addenbrooke's Cognitive Examination (MACE) [25] and the Montreal Cognitive Assessment (MoCA) [46], were examined in counterbalanced fashion in a screening test accuracy study [33] using cut-offs from the index studies of the tests (MACE $\leq$25/30; MoCA <26/30).

In the study population (N = 260), 182 had MACE scores $\leq$25/30 and 192 had MoCA scores <26/30. Constructing a 2 × 2 table, the values for a, b, c, and d were 164, 28, 18, and 50 respectively.

Hence observed agreement was:

$$
\begin{aligned}
P_a &= (a+d)/N \\
&= (164+50)/260 \\
&= 0.823
\end{aligned}
$$

Agreement expected by chance was:

$$
\begin{aligned}
P_c &= (a+b)(a+c)/N^2 + (c+d)(b+d)/N^2 \\
&= (164+28)(164+18)/260^2 + (18+50)(28+50)/260^2 \\
&= 0.517+0.078 \\
&= 0.595
\end{aligned}
$$

Therefore:

$$
\begin{aligned}
\kappa &= (P_a - P_c)/(1-P_c) \\
&= (0.823-0.595)/(1-0.595) \\
&= 0.563
\end{aligned}
$$

Based on the convention of Landis and Koch [30], this value of κ would be interpreted as moderate agreement (>0.4–0.6) (Larner, unpublished observations).

Kappa can be extended to encompass more than two categories and more than two raters, in which case some form of weighting may be required [16, 21].

In certain circumstances, kappa and Matthews' correlation coefficient (MCC; Sect. 4.5) coincide (symmetric matrix) [17], although these circumstances are unlikely to occur in clinical practice. Delgado and Tibau characterized kappa as the harmonic mean of the Youden index (Y; Sect. 4.2) and predictive summary index (PSI; Sect. 4.3) in this particular situation [17] (Sect. 4.4).

**Worked Example: Kappa Statistic as Harmonic Mean of Y and PSI**

In the screening test accuracy study of MACE [35], at the MACE cut-off of ≤20/30 the value of Y was 0.619 (Sect. 4.2) and of PSI was 0.334 (Sect. 4.3). If the kappa statistic is calculated as the harmonic mean of Y and PSI (Sect. 4.4), then:

$$\begin{aligned}
\kappa &= 2/\left[1/Y + 1/PSI\right] \\
&= 2.Y.PSI/(Y+PSI) \\
&= 2 \times 0.619 \times 0.334/(0.619+0.334) \\
&= 0.413/0.953 \\
&= 0.433
\end{aligned}$$

Note that this result does not agree with the calculation of "Accuracy with kappa statistic" (= 0.378) above, nor with the "unbiased Acc" (= 0.378) shown in Sect. 3.2.4. However, if the equation for kappa is re-written as:

$$\kappa = 2(ad-bc)/\left[(a+c)(b+d)+(a+b)(c+d)\right]$$

then using the data from the MACE study where a (=TP) = 104, b (=FP) = 188, c (=FN) = 10, and d (=TN) = 453, we obtain:

$$\begin{aligned}
\kappa &= 2(ad-bc)/\left[(a+c)(b+d)+(a+b)(c+d)\right] \\
&= 2 \times 45232/\left[(114 \times 641)+(292 \times 463)\right] \\
&= 2 \times 45232/73074+135196 \\
&= 90464/208270 \\
&= 0.434
\end{aligned}$$

[The different results relate to rounding errors.]

Hence the different result of "kappa statistic as harmonic mean of Y and PSI" compared to "Accuracy with kappa statistic" and "unbiased Acc" is a consequence of the different marginal totals. In the situation where b = c (i.e. a symmetric matrix) then the results would align, and would also be equal to the Matthews' correlation coefficient (Sect. 4.5).

Kappa statistic has shortcomings. It is affected by prevalence, and hence comparisons of its value determined in different populations may not be appropriate. As mentioned, it is also affected by class imbalance, when kappa scores may be low even when observed agreement is high. Moreover, kappa does not distinguish between types and sources of disagreement. It has been argued that the proportion of specific agreement, expressing the agreement separately for positive and negative ratings, is more clinically informative [18]. The first of these measures is identical to the F measure or Dice coefficient (Sect. 4.9). Some advocate that kappa should be avoided altogether [17]. Perhaps HMYPSI (Sect. 4.4) might be preferred, as it is an absolute measure rather than a relative measure.

### 7.2.3   Limits of Agreement: Bland-Altman Method

Limits of agreement are not related to the 2 × 2 contingency table and are included here for completeness, in order to contrast with the previously described Cohen's kappa "measure of agreement". This is a method to provide a measure of agreement between tests by estimating how far apart the two values are on average and putting an interval around this [7]. The findings may be illustrated in a Bland-Altman plot of difference between test scores against their mean. The limits of agreement thus defined indicate how closely two methods agree, but what is accepted as "close" remains a clinical rather than a statistical judgement. The Bland-Altman methodology is a simple way to evaluate bias between mean differences which avoids the potentially erroneous conclusions based on correlation analyses.

## 7.3   Other Tables

### 7.3.1   Higher Order Tables

As previously discussed (Sect. 1.5), setting a decision threshold or dichotomisation point is critical to the construction of a 2 × 2 contingency table (potential methods for doing this are discussed in Sects. 6.2.1, 6.2.2, 6.2.3, 6.2.4, 6.2.5, and 6.2.6). This is not always a straightforward process. In clinical practice, dichotomisation may be inappropriate, for example when the object of tests is something other than simply identifying the presence or absence of disease. Furthermore, in screening or diagnostic test accuracy studies patients may not be tested with either the diagnostic test or the reference standard, or values may be lost or indeterminate. To accommodate the vagaries of real world practice, it may be more appropriate to use larger contingency tables, such as 2 × 3 [52], 2 × 4 [14], or 3 × 3 ([51], p. 31), although this complicates the calculation of any of the measures previously discussed.

### 7.3.2   Interval Likelihood Ratios (ILRs)

An example of a higher order table may be provided by the use of interval likelihood ratios [12], as opposed to the more usual dichotomisation into positive and negative likelihood ratios (Sect. 2.3.4). Selecting the intervals is somewhat arbitrary, and the smaller the numbers in each interval the wider the confidence intervals (Sect. 1.7) are likely to be.

**Fig. 7.1** MACE scores (x axis) by patient diagnosis (N = 755). (Adapted from [35])

**Worked Example: Higher Order Tables – Interval Likelihood Ratios**
In the screening test accuracy study of MACE [35], category-specific positive and negative likelihood ratios were calculated at the MACE cut-off ≤20/30, such that LR+ = 3.11 and LR− = 0.124 at this cut-off (Sect. 2.3.4). However, looking at the spread of MACE scores in the whole patient study cohort (N = 755), as shown in Fig. 7.1, the overlap between dementia and no dementia patients extended over a range of MACE scores.

Although category-specific LRs may be calculated for each cut-off [35], another approach would be to calculate interval LRs (ILRs). Hence, a 2 × 5 table was constructed, from which ILRs were calculated, as TPR/FPR, or as $p$(T+ | D+)/$p$(T+ | D−), as shown:

| MACE score/30 | Diagnosis: Dementia | Diagnosis: No dementia | Interval Likelihood Ratio (ILR) |
|---|---|---|---|
| 26–30 | 1 | 202 | (1/114)/(202/641) = 0.028 |
| 21–25 | 9 | 251 | (9/114)/(251/641) = 0.202 |
| 16–20 | 29 | 121 | (29/114)/(121/641) = 1.348 |
| 11–15 | 40 | 52 | (40/114)/(52/641) = 4.325 |
| ≤10 | 35 | 15 | (35/114)/(15/641) = 13.12 |
| **TOTAL** | **114** | **641** | |

The ILR for MACE scores in the interval 26–30/30 was very small, 0.028, suggesting a very large change in probability (see Table 2.1 for a qualitative classification of LR values) and hence diagnostic gain for a diagnosis of no dementia. Likewise for the interval ≤10/30 the LR value, 13.12, was very large for a diagnosis of dementia. For the intervals 21–25/30 and 11–15/30 the LR values were qualitatively only moderate, although it should be noted that they represent an approximate change in probability of +/−25% (Table 2.1). The LR for the interval 16–20/30 was close to unity, suggesting only slight change in probability, and hence no diagnostic gain. This contrasts with the finding when the test was simply dichotomised at the cut-off ≤20/30. Results falling near a dichotomous cut-off may be distorted. The information from ILRs may assist clinical decision making to a greater extent than the simple dichotomised values for LR+ and LR− (Larner, unpublished observations).

## 7.3.3   Three-Way Classification (Trichotomisation)

As previously mentioned (Sect. 1.6), three-way classification, or trichotomisation, is a method which may permit better classification accuracy by excluding or deselecting uncertain test scores, usually those falling near a dichotomous cut-off (Sect. 7.3.2), which are most error-prone. Unclassified individuals or instances may then require further assessment for correct classification. A downside of this approach is that calculation of sensitivity and specificity becomes cumbersome, being meant for dichotomous classification [31].

**Worked Example: Three-Way Classification (Trichotomisation)**
In the screening test accuracy study of MACE [35], result-specific likelihood ratios were calculated at all MACE cut-offs and plotted (Fig. 7.2).

If LR values >0.5 and <2 are considered to produce only a "slight" (decrease or increase respectively) in the probability of disease, whereas values ≤0.5 or ≥2 produce moderate change (Table 2.1), the former range might be deemed a zone of uncertainty. From the calculations and the plot it is possible to read off the range of MACE test scores corresponding to this range of LRs, namely ≤16/30 to ≤21/30 (the LR value at 18/30 is outside the 0.5<LR<2 range, but it is included here for convenience). This range contains 25.9% of all scores (196/755) and has an interval LR of (33/114)/(163/641) = 1.14. At the optimal MACE cut-off of ≤20/30, this range contains 63.1% of all the errors (4/10 false negatives, 121/188 false positives) (Larner, unpublished observations).

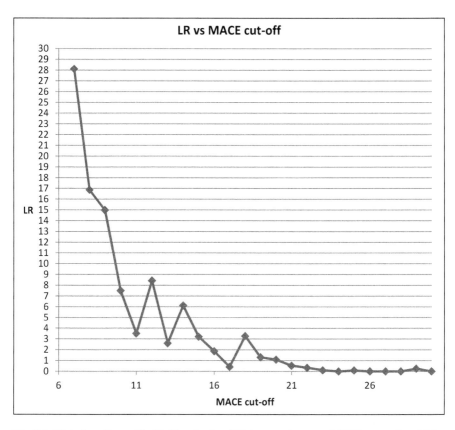

**Fig. 7.2** Plot of result-specific likelihood ratios (LRs) on y axis versus MACE scores (x axis) for dementia diagnosis. (Data from [35]). Below MACE cut-off 6/30, LR values tend to ∞

## 7.3.4   Combining Test Results

If some results are uncertain, requiring further tests for correct classification, then methods to combine test scores may be required. As previously mentioned in passing (Sect. 2.3.4), calculation of likelihood ratios provides a method for combining the results of multiple tests (1,2,…n), assuming the conditional independence of the tests in the presence and absence of the target diagnosis, by using Bayes' formula such that:

$$\text{Post-test odds} \quad = \quad \text{Pre-test odds} \times LR_1 \times LR_2 \times \ldots LR_n$$

**Worked Example: Combining Tests: MACE and SMC Likert Scale (1)**
In the screening test accuracy study of MACE [35], some patients (N = 129) were also administered a single-item cognitive screening question, the Subjective Memory Complaint (SMC) Likert Scale [49], in order to assess whether combining a patient-performance cognitive screener (MACE) with subjective memory evaluation (SMC Likert Scale) gave additional diagnostic information [34].

In the SMC Likert Scale, participants are asked: "In general, how would you rate your memory?" and given a choice of five possible responses: 1 = poor; 2 = fair; 3 = good; 4 = very good; 5 = excellent. SMC Likert Scale scores may be easily dichotomised: a score of 1 or 2 is categorised as SMC+, scores >2 as SMC− (i.e. higher scores better) [49].

60 of the 129 patients administered both tests, MACE and SMC Likert Scale, received a clinical diagnosis of cognitive impairment, hence pre-test probability (prevalence) of cognitive impairment in this cohort was 0.465, and pre-test odds were 0.869. Pre-test probability against disease was 69/129 = 0.535, and pre-test odds against disease were (1 − 0.465)/0.465 = 1.15 (see Sect. 1.3.3).

Using the MACE cut-off of ≤25/30 for cognitive impairment, established in the index study [25], LR+ for a diagnosis of cognitive impairment was $p(R_i | D+)/p(R_i | D−) = (54/60)/(44/69) = 1.41$, a value producing only a slight increase in the probability of disease (Table 2.1). LR− for a diagnosis of no cognitive impairment was (6/60)/(25/69) = 0.276, a value producing a moderate increase in the probability of no disease (Table 2.1).

Using the SMC Likert Scale cut-off of ≤2, LR+ for a diagnosis of cognitive impairment was $p(R_i | D+)/p(R_i | D−) = (42/60)/(60/69) = 0.805$, suggesting that subjective evaluation of memory actually slightly decreased the probability of a diagnosis of cognitive impairment (it increases the probability of a diagnosis of functional cognitive disorder [6, 39]). LR− for a diagnosis of no cognitive impairment was (18/60)/(9/69) = 2.3, a value producing a moderate decrease in the probability of no disease (Table 2.1).

The results of the two tests were combined using Bayes' formula:

$$
\begin{aligned}
\text{Post-test odds} &= \text{Pre-test odds} \times \text{LR+}_{\text{MACE}} \times \text{LR+}_{\text{SMC}} \\
&= 0.869 \times 1.41 \times 0.805 \\
&= 0.986
\end{aligned}
$$

This can be converted back to a post-test-probability using the equation:

$$
\begin{aligned}
\text{Post-test probability} &= \text{Post-test odds} / (1 + \text{post-test odds}) \\
&= 0.986 / (1 + 0.986) \\
&= 0.496
\end{aligned}
$$

Thus, this combination of tests shows only a marginal improvement over the pre-test probability (0.465).

It is also possible to calculate the combined odds against disease using Bayes' formula:

$$
\begin{aligned}
\text{Post-test odds against} \; &= \; \text{Pre-test odds against} \times \text{LR-}_{\text{MACE}} \times \text{LR-}_{\text{SMC}} \\
&= \; 1.15 \times 0.276 \times 2.3 \\
&= \; 0.73
\end{aligned}
$$

This can be converted back to a post-test-probability against disease using the equation:

$$
\begin{aligned}
\text{Post-test probability against} \; &= \; 1/(1 + \text{post-test odds against}) \\
&= \; 1/(1 + 0.73) \\
&= \; 0.578
\end{aligned}
$$

Thus, this combination of tests shows a marginal increase over the pre-test probability against disease (0.535) (Larner, unpublished observations).

This Bayesian approach to combining test results may be compared with combination using simple logical rules ([36], p. 81–2, 133–6), or Boolean operators.

Using simple logical rules, one may construct tables akin to the truth tables developed for use in logic by Wittgenstein for the "and" and "or" connectives used to determine the truth or falsity of simple propositions (Fig. 7.3)

The Bayesian approach may also be compared with Boolean operators, after George Boole (1815–64), specifically combination using the "AND" rule, where both tests are required to be positive for the target diagnosis to be made (i.e. any combination other than both tests positive is considered to rule out the diagnosis, an approach which privileges identification of true and false positives; Fig. 7.3a). This is sometimes known as series, serial or conjunctive combination, "believe the negative", or sequency (the first of these terms is avoided here as ambiguous, sometimes being used to refer to the situation where performance of a second test is dependent on the outcome of the first test, rather than all tests being performed on all subjects regardless of the result of the first).

Another Boolean operator, or method of combination, is the "OR" rule, also known as parallel or compensatory combination, "believe the positive", or simultaneity (i.e. any combination other than both tests negative is considered to rule in the diagnosis, an approach which privileges identification of true and false negatives; Fig. 7.3b). (The Boolean operator "NOT" applies to the paired logical complementary measures or negations considered in Chapter 3.)

Evidently the "AND" criterion is more severe, and preferable if FP outcomes are particularly to be avoided, whilst the "OR" criterion is more liberal and preferable if FN outcomes are particularly undesirable.

a) "and"

| Classifier diagnosis | | | |
|---|---|---|---|
| **Test 1** | **Test 2** | **Test 3** | **Test 1 "and" Test 2** |
| D+ | D+ | – | D+ |
| D+ | D– | – | D– |
| D– | D+ | – | D– |
| D– | D– | – | D– |
|  |  |  | **"and" Test 3** |
| D+ | D+ | D+ | D+ |
| D+ | D+ | D– | D– |
| D+ | D– | D+ | D– |
| D– | D+ | D+ | D– |
| D+ | D– | D– | D– |
| D– | D+ | D– | D– |
| D– | D– | D+ | D– |
| D– | D– | D– | D– |

b) "or"

| Classifier diagnosis | | | |
|---|---|---|---|
| **Test 1** | **Test 2** | **Test 3** | **Test 1 "or" Test 2** |
| D+ | D+ | – | D+ |
| D+ | D– | – | D+ |
| D– | D+ | – | D+ |
| D– | D– | – | D– |
|  |  |  | **"or" Test 3** |
| D+ | D+ | D+ | D+ |
| D+ | D+ | D– | D+ |
| D+ | D– | D+ | D+ |
| D– | D+ | D+ | D+ |
| D+ | D– | D– | D+ |
| D– | D+ | D– | D+ |
| D– | D– | D+ | D+ |
| D– | D– | D– | D– |

**Fig. 7.3** Truth tables for simple logical rules of combination for 2 or 3 tests: (**a**) "and"; (**b**) "or"

**Worked Example: Combining Tests: MACE and SMC Likert Scale (2)**
MACE and SMC Likert results were combined in series: both tests were required to be positive (MACE $\leq 25/30$ and SMC $\leq 2$) for the target diagnosis of cognitive impairment to be made. This permitted the construction of a $2 \times 2$ contingency table accommodating both tests (Fig. 7.4a).

From the combined contingency table, the positive predictive value may be calculated as TP/(TP + FP) = 40/(40 + 40) = 0.5, similar to the post-test-probability value obtained using the Bayesian method based on multiplication of pre-test odds and individual test LRs (0.496).

The negative predictive value may be calculated as TN/(FN + TN) = 29/(20 + 29) = 0.59, similar to the post-test-probability against (0.578) (Larner, unpublished observations).

**Fig. 7.4**  2 × 2 contingency tables for combination of Mini-Addenbrooke's Cognitive Examination (MACE) and SMC Likert Scale outcomes (N = 129) for the diagnosis of cognitive impairment: (**a**) "AND" rule, series combination; (**b**) "OR" rule, parallel combination. (Data from [34])

a)

| | | **Diagnosis** | |
| --- | --- | --- | --- |
| | | **Cognitive impairment present** | **Cognitive impairment absent** |
| **MACE "AND" SMC outcome** | ≤25/30 and ≤2 | True positive [TP] = 40 | False positive [FP] = 40 |
| | ≤25/30 and >2, or >25/30 | False negative, [FN] = 20 | True negative [TN] = 29 |

b)

| | | **Diagnosis** | |
| --- | --- | --- | --- |
| | | **Cognitive impairment present** | **Cognitive impairment absent** |
| **MACE "OR" SMC outcome** | ≤25/30 or ≤2 | True positive [TP] = 56 | False positive [FP] = 64 |
| | >25/30 and >2 | False negative [FN] = 4 | True negative [TN] = 5 |

It is also possible to calculate Sens and Spec for two tests (Test 1, Test 2) applied in series ("AND") or in parallel ("OR") based on individual test Sens and Spec using the equations:

$$\text{Sens}_{1\text{"AND"}2} = \text{Sens}_1 \times \text{Sens}_2$$

$$\begin{aligned}\text{Spec}_{1\text{"AND"}2} &= \text{Spec}_1 + \left[(1 - \text{Spec}_1) \times \text{Spec}_2\right] \\ &= \text{Spec}_1 + \text{Spec}_2 - \left[\text{Spec}_1 \times \text{Spec}_2\right]\end{aligned}$$

$$\begin{aligned}\text{Sens}_{1\text{"OR"}2} &= \text{Sens}_1 + \left[(1 - \text{Sens}_1) \times \text{Sens}_2\right] \\ &= \text{Sens}_1 + \text{Sens}_2 - \left[\text{Sens}_1 \times \text{Sens}_2\right]\end{aligned}$$

$$\text{Spec}_{1\text{"OR"}2} = \text{Spec}_1 \times \text{Spec}_2$$

**Worked Example: Combining Tests: MACE and SMC Likert Scale (3)**

Sens and Spec for the combination of MACE and SMC Likert results were calculated for the "AND" and "OR" combinations.

For the "AND" combination:

$$\begin{aligned} \text{Sens}_{\text{MACE"AND"SMC}} &= \text{Sens}_{\text{MACE}} \times \text{Sens}_{\text{SMC}} \\ &= 0.70 \times 0.90 \\ &= 0.63 \end{aligned}$$

$$\begin{aligned} \text{Spec}_{\text{MACE"AND"SMC}} &= \text{Spec}_{\text{MACE}} + \left[ (1 - \text{Spec}_{\text{MACE}}) \times \text{Spec}_{\text{SMC}} \right] \\ &= 0.13 + [0.87 \times 0.36] \\ &= 0.44 \end{aligned}$$

Looking at the 2 × 2 contingency table for series combination of MACE and SMC Likert (Figure 7.3a), $\text{Sens}_{\text{MACE"AND"SMC}} = \text{TP}/(\text{TP} + \text{FN}) = 40/60 = 0.67$, and $\text{Spec}_{\text{MACE"AND"SMC}} = \text{TN}/(\text{FP} + \text{TN}) = 29/69 = 0.42$, both results similar to the above calculations.

For the "OR" combination:

$$\begin{aligned} \text{Sens}_{\text{MACE"OR"SMC}} &= \text{Sens}_{\text{MACE}} + \left[ (1 - \text{Sens}_{\text{MACE}}) \times \text{Sens}_{\text{SMC}} \right] \\ &= 0.70 + [0.30 \times 0.90] \\ &= 0.97 \end{aligned}$$

$$\begin{aligned} \text{Spec}_{\text{MACE"OR"SMC}} &= \text{Spec}_{\text{MACE}} \times \text{Spec}_{\text{SMC}} \\ &= 0.13 \times 0.36 \\ &= 0.05 \end{aligned}$$

Looking at the 2 × 2 contingency table for parallel combination of MACE and SMC Likert (Fig. 7.4b), $\text{Sens}_{\text{MACE"OR"SMC}} = \text{TP}/(\text{TP} + \text{FN}) = 54/60 = 0.93$, and $\text{Spec}_{\text{MACE"OR"SMC}} = \text{TN}/(\text{FP} + \text{TN}) = 5/69 = 0.07$, both results similar to the above calculations (Larner, unpublished observations).

These two approaches, Bayesian and Boolean, to combining test results have also been examined for another pair of screening tests [44].

**Worked Example: Combining Tests: AD8 and 6CIT**

In the assessment of cognitive complaints, some authorities recommend the use of both a patient performance measurement and an informant interview before making a diagnosis of dementia. A previous study [32] in a dedicated cognitive disorders clinic examined both the informant AD8 scale [23] and the Six-item Cognitive Impairment Test (6CIT) patient performance cognitive screening instrument [11]. Both of these tests are negatively scored (i.e. higher scores = impairment worse).

51 of the 177 patients administered both tests were diagnosed with dementia based on clinical diagnostic criteria, hence pre-test probability (prevalence) of dementia in this cohort was 0.288, and pre-test odds (Sect. 1.3.3) was 0.405.

Using the AD8 cut-off of $\geq 2/8$, LR+ for a diagnosis of dementia was $p(R_i \mid D+)/p(R_i \mid D-) = (49/51)/(112/126) = 1.08$, a value producing only a slight increase in the probability of dementia (Table 2.1), notwithstanding its very high sensitivity.

Using the 6CIT cut-off of $\geq 8/28$, LR+ for a diagnosis of dementia was $p(R_i \mid D+)/p(R_i \mid D-) = (44/51)/(48/126) = 2.26$, a value producing a moderate increase in the probability of dementia (Table 2.1).

The results of the two tests were combined using Bayes' formula:

$$
\begin{aligned}
\text{Post-test odds} &= \text{Pre-test odds} \times \text{LR}_{AD8} \times \text{LR}_{6CIT} \\
&= 0.405 \times 1.08 \times 2.26 \\
&= 0.988
\end{aligned}
$$

This can be converted back to a post-test-probability using the equation:

$$
\begin{aligned}
\text{Post-test probability} &= \text{Post-test odds} / (1 + \text{post-test odds}) \\
&= 0.988 / (1 + 0.988) \\
&= 0.497
\end{aligned}
$$

This combination of tests therefore shows improvement compared to the pre-test probability of 0.288.

The Bayesian approach to combining test results may be compared with combination using the simple logical "AND" rule (series combination or sequency): both tests were required to be positive (AD8 $\geq 2/8$ and 6CIT $\geq 8/28$) for the target diagnosis of dementia to be made. This permitted the construction of a $2 \times 2$ contingency table accommodating both tests (Fig. 7.5).

From the contingency table, the positive predictive value may be calculated as TP/(TP + FP) = 42/(42 + 45) = 0.483, similar to the post-test-probability value obtained using the Bayesian method based on multiplication of pre-test odds and individual test LRs (Larner, unpublished observations).

**Fig. 7.5** 2 × 2 contingency table for series combination of informant Ascertain Dementia 8 (AD8) "AND" Six-item Cognitive Impairment Test (6CIT) outcomes (N = 177) for the diagnosis of dementia. (Data updated from [32])

| | | Diagnosis | |
|---|---|---|---|
| | | **Dementia present** | **Dementia absent** |
| AD8 "AND" 6CIT outcome | ≥2/8 and ≥8/28 | True positive [TP] = 42 | False positive [FP] = 45 |
| | ≥2/8 and >8/28, or <2/8 | False negative [FN] = 9 | True negative [TN] = 81 |

Generally, sequential combination of tests leads to improvement in specificity, false positive rate, positive predictive value, and positive likelihood ratio. Conversely, sensitivity, false negative rate, negative predictive value and negative likelihood ratio are generally inferior with this method of combination ([36], p. 81–2, 133–6; [41], p. 119–43).

One possible advantage of the sequence method over the Bayesian method is that it requires construction of a new 2 × 2 contingency table and hence the opportunity to calculate many of the outcome measures discussed in previous chapters of this book for the combination of tests, not only post-test probability. For example, it is immediately evident (Fig. 7.5) that the combination of AD8 and 6CIT is sensitive for dementia diagnosis (0.82) with a high negative predictive value (0.90).

When more than two tests are involved, the Bayesian approach of multiplying the pre-test odds by the individual LR values may become easier to apply than constructing new 2 × 2 tables. However, this may conceal some shortcomings of combining tests.

---

**Worked Example: Combining Tests: The Triple Test**

The Attended With sign (AW), the Applause Sign (AS), and the Head-Turning Sign (HTS), have individually been noted as possible clinical markers of the presence of cognitive impairment. Their combination as the "Triple Test" to detect cognitive impairment has been suggested [26] and this has been examined [38].

Of 85 patients administered all three tests, 44 were diagnosed with cognitive impairment based on clinical diagnostic criteria, hence pre-test probability (prevalence) of cognitive impairment in this cohort was 0.52, and pre-test odds (Sect. 1.3.3) was 1.07.

LR+ for each sign was as follows (unpublished observations from data in [36]): $LR_{AW}$ = 2.07; $LR_{AS}$ = 2.08; and $LR_{HTS}$ = 11.33.

The results of the three tests were combined:

$$
\begin{aligned}
\text{Post-test odds} &= \text{Pre-test odds} \times LR_{AW} \times LR_{AS} \times LR_{HTS} \\
&= 1.07 \times 2.07 \times 2.08 \times 11.33 \\
&= 52.19
\end{aligned}
$$

This can be converted back to a post-test-probability using the equation:

$$
\begin{aligned}
\text{Post-test probability} &= \text{Post-test odds} / (1 + \text{post-test odds}) \\
&= 52.20 / (1 + 52.20) \\
&= 0.998
\end{aligned}
$$

This combination of tests, the Triple Test, therefore shows a positive predictive value of 1, a marked improvement compared to the pre-test probability (0.52).

However, it may not be immediately evident from this approach, but clear from the 2 × 2 contingency table (Fig. 7.6), that although both the PPV and specificity are perfect, the NPV is poor (0.5) and the sensitivity is negligible (0.07), with many false negatives, a pattern to be expected with the sequential combination of tests (Larner, unpublished observations). Many clinicians would find such test sensitivity unfit for purpose. The truth table for three tests combined using the "and" connective (Fig. 7.3a) also indicates the likelihood of many false negatives since so many of the outcomes are classified as negative.

**Fig. 7.6**  2 × 2 contingency table for Triple Test (series combination of AW "AND" AS "AND" HTS) (N = 85) for the diagnosis of cognitive impairment. (Data from [38]). See also Fig. 7.3a.

| AW, AS, "AND" HTS outcome | | Diagnosis | |
|---|---|---|---|
| | | **Cognitive impairment present** | **Cognitive impairment absent** |
| | **All tests positive** | True positive [TP] = 3 | False positive [FP] = 0 |
| | **Any one negative** | False negative [FN] = 41 | True negative [TN] = 41 |

## 7.3.5   Decision Trees; Machine Learning

As these examples have shown, clinical problems may often be defined as staged processes consisting of successive dichotomous actions, concordant with the mode of clinical practice. Sequential testing strategies may be conveniently structured in the form of a decision tree.

Decision trees represent the chronological order of events with probabilities assigned to outcomes denoted by chance nodes (circles), to model uncertain events, and decision nodes (squares). Decision trees should incorporate all possible options (e.g. actions which may be chosen, or outcomes which may occur with each option) and hence extend beyond binary classification. Decision trees may be useful for the development of both diagnostic and prognostic predictions in the form of decision rules and algorithms. Such algorithms may permit standardization of approach, but may risk stifling innovation.

A clinical example is the cognitive disorders examination or Codex, a two-step decision tree for diagnostic prediction which incorporates results of two sequential tests (three-word recall and spatial orientation followed by a simplified clock drawing test) resulting in four terminal nodes with different probabilities of dementia diagnosis [5, 57]. Other screening instruments may be reformulated as decision trees [40].

The data of the MACE and SMC Likert Scale study [34] (Sect. 7.3.4 and Fig. 7.4a) may be reformatted as a simple decision tree (Fig. 7.7). Following the root node of "suspected cognitive impairment", the administration of tests is denoted by chance nodes (circles), modelling uncertain outcomes, with the continuous input variables collapsed into two categories according to test cut-off. Classifier diagnosis is denoted by decision nodes (squares), in this instance forming the terminal or leaf nodes of the tree. Decision trees may be arranged running from left to right, or from top to bottom, with the latter preferred here so that the terminal nodes may be seen to correspond to the rows of the $2 \times 2$ contingency table, both denoting classifier diagnosis (compare with Fig. 7.4a).

Decision trees may incorporate either absolute numbers or probabilities (see Fig. 7.7a, b respectively for the MACE "AND" SMC Likert Scale). That the order of tests gives the same classification is evident (Fig. 7.7c, an inversion of Fig. 7.7a), and the "OR" combination can also be represented (Fig. 7.7d).

Although not part of typical decision trees, more distal "branches" or "leaves" have been added to these figures to show criterion diagnoses for comparison with the classifier diagnoses, information which permits summation of TP, FP, FN, and TN and hence construction of "AND" and "OR" $2 \times 2$ contingency tables (Fig. 7.4).

Each path or route through the decision tree represents a classification decision rule, which may be characterised by "if-then" rules or conditional statements: if condition 1 and condition 2 occur, then a specified outcome occurs. For example, in Fig. 7.7, if MACE $\leq 25/30$ and SMC = 1–2, then classifier diagnosis is cognitive impairment. If MACE $\leq 25/30$ and SMC = 3–5 then, according to one classification rule, classifier diagnosis is no cognitive impairment (Fig. 7.7a), whereas following

**a) "AND" absolute numbers**

**b) "AND" probabilities**

**Fig. 7.7** Decision trees for combination of Mini-Addenbrooke's Cognitive Examination (MACE) and SMC Likert Scale outcomes (N = 129) for the diagnosis of cognitive impairment (data from [34]): (**a**) "AND" absolute numbers; (**b**) "AND" probabilities; (**c**) "AND" tree inverted; (**d**) "OR" absolute numbers (an extra, detached, set of leaves denoting criterion diagnoses has been added in each case to permit easy calculation of TP, FP, FN, and TN numbers)

a different classification rule, classifier diagnosis is cognitive impairment (Fig. 7.7d). In this particular instance, these two rules happen to be equivalent to the "AND" and "OR" Boolean classifiers.

Binary decision tree methodology may be used to segment test groups into meaningful subgroups according to certain variables that may encompass a predictive value, for example using a Classification and Regression Tree (CART) [10]. Other algorithms are available to develop decision trees and may be found in data mining software [53].

Machine learning ("artificial intelligence") classifiers "learn" to predict outcome based on large sets of variables. Support vector machines are typically used for binary classification whilst neural networks can map a large number of possible

**c) "AND" tree inverted**

**d) "OR" absolute numbers**

**Fig. 7.7** (continued)

outcomes. Variables are projected to high dimensional space (one variable mapped to one dimension); the classifier is the hyperplane which separates the data points, a line in two dimensions, a surface in three dimensions. This may be straight or flat with linear hyperplane solutions, curvy or rippled if non-linear (with risk of overfitting). The suggestion (Sect. 1.7) that 2 × 2 table outcomes might be explored in 4-dimensional space might be susceptible to such methods.

Machine learning methods are unbiased and very sensitive. Large amounts of data are needed to build reliable classification, using a training dataset to train the classifier, and validation. Measures such as accuracy, AUC ROC, F measure, and a test of significance (producing a *p* value) are often used to evaluate the quality of such classification models.

Whether these methods can be brought to effective use in clinical diagnosis remains to be seen [13]. Diagnostic classifiers are not yet in regular clinical use; human judgment currently prevails.

## 7.3.6   Fourfold Pattern of Risk Attitudes

Tversky and Kahneman noted that "the most distinctive implication of prospect theory is the fourfold pattern of risk attitudes" ([56], p.306). Essentially this is a 2 × 2 contingency table cross-classifying gains and losses as classes against high and low probabilities as potential classifiers (Fig. 7.8). To preserve benefits, one may be risk averse for gains, whereas to avoid harms one may be risk seeking for losses. The fourfold pattern has applications in many fields, including economics and law, and is relevant to the net harm to net benefit (H/B) ratio (described in Sect. 2.3.5).

## 7.3.7   Epistemological Matrix

"What do I know?" asked Montaigne (1533-92). Do we know, or simply think we know? Is there an objective knowledge, which we may only perceive subjectively, as through a prism, through the medium of the workings of our brain? "We do not look at things as they are, but as we are" said Kant (1724–1804).

Such reflections might also be summarised in a 2 × 2 table, which I venture to call an epistemological matrix (Fig. 7.9), and which may have relevance not only to that sphere of philosophy (as all knowledge is historically contingent) but also to

**Fig. 7.8** The fourfold pattern of risk attitudes

**Fig. 7.9** The (2 × 2) epistemological matrix

psychology. It takes uncertainty as inherent to the human condition, with marked class imbalance due to the predominance of the unknown column, and to the unknown unknown category in particular. We are blind to our blindness, and have an almost unlimited ability to ignore our ignorance ([28], p. 24, 201); "unobservables cannot be detected, and are epistemically unavailable" [55]. Consider the experiential and intellectual limitations of the residents of Edwin Abbott's two-dimensional *Flatland* (even the pentagonal doctors!). Here one might also include the anoetic or nonknowing consciousness proposed by Tulving, encompassing abilities such as implicit memory (we all have a degree of cognitive anosognosia). The omniscient lies outside the matrix.

## 7.4   Conclusion: Which Measure(s) Should Be Used?

> As in any sorting-out process, Roget was plagued by the big problem inherent in classification: the validity of categories vs. the continuum of nature ([20], p. 268).

As I have learned more over the years, I have been intrigued by the number of measures which may be derived from an ostensibly simple $2 \times 2$ grid (and have added to this number: CDI+, CDI−, Sect. 2.4.2; HMYPSI, Sect. 4.4; SUI, SDI, Sect. 4.10; LDM, LPM, Sect. 5.5; NNSU, NNSD, Sect. 5.7), and by their interrelationships. The analysis offered in this book has been restricted, in the interests of simplicity and by the author's limited abilities, to binary classification. This is recognised to have shortcomings (e.g. loss of information, Sects. 1.5, 1.6, and 7.3.1; misclassification, Sect. 3.2.5) and potential solutions (e.g. higher order tables, Sect. 7.3.2; trichotomisation, Sects. 1.6 and 7.3.3) although these may not be straightforward to apply. Moreover, correct construction of $2 \times 2$ tables and calculation of outputs does not obviate the necessity to assess risk of bias (internal validity) and generalisability of findings (external validity). However, in medical practice, dichotomisation is pragmatic for clinical decision making [22], and hence likely to continue.

How, then, should one steer a course through the many summary measures which have been described in this text? What metric(s) should be selected for analysis of a study? This may depend in part on the particular question being asked, the context, and also familiarity, personal preference (what one finds most intuitive, or easily communicable to patients) and fashion. In clinical medicine the F measure and Matthews' correlation coefficient are seldom used [37, 42] whereas the former is almost obligatory in information retrieval and machine learning contexts despite its shortcomings [50].

The outputs of meta-analyses are usually given in terms of summary sensitivity and specificity and ROC curve but, as has been pointed out [22], these measures do not answer clinicians' questions, being orientated to the test rather than to the patient. Predictive values, being orientated to the patient, might seem more clinically useful but these values are unstable because of their dependence on prevalence. Positive and negative likelihood ratios may obviate these problems, but dichotomisation risks loss of information and distortion, and calculation of interval likelihood ratios is more involved and the choice of intervals may be arbitrary.

As stated in the Introductory chapter (Sect. 1.7), it might be intuited that the very multiplicity of the measures which may be derived from $2 \times 2$ contingency tables suggests their inadequacy, if summary statistics reduce the information to a single characteristic of the data. Is there a minimum set or a standard "dashboard" [54], a limited set of metrics which shows what "really matters" (i.e. guides what we do) and hence which might be agreed by expert consensus? None yet exist, to my knowledge. Both the STAndards for the Reporting of Diagnostic accuracy studies guideline (STARD [9]) and its iteration for studies in dementia (STARDdem [48]) recommend sensitivity and specificity as keywords of papers reporting diagnostic test accuracy studies. Likelihood ratios may be used as the basis for recommendations about suitable tests (e.g. for dementia [47]). Some measures may be preferred as test-oriented (Sens, Spec, FPR, FNR, LRs), or patient-oriented (PPV, NPV, predictive ratios), or as indices of validity (LR, DOR, Y), or as more intuitive (Net reclassification improvement, "Number needed to" measures). Test shortcomings, as evidenced by the use of error notation (Sect. 1.4) wherever appropriate throughout this book, may also be denoted by what I have ventured to term "metrics of limitation" [43] such as false rates (positive, negative, discovery, reassurance; Sects. 2.2.3 and 2.3.3), misclassification rate (Sect. 3.2.5), net harm to net benefit (H/B) ratio (Sect. 2.3.5), likelihood to be diagnosed or misdiagnosed (Sect. 5.5), and clinical disutility indexes (Sect. 2.4.2). Other metrics may be less familiar, and outside clinician literacy, but this could be addressed if the measures were deemed sufficiently useful, for example in communicating information to patients. Ultimately, the provision of test datasets should allow researchers to calculate any parameter of interest not explicitly stated in the index paper.

"Ars longa vita brevis" wrote Hippocrates (or one of his followers). The art of medicine may be, for the gifted, an intuitive process, but for others the art is long and deliberative. Intuitive thinking may be liable to error [28]. The use of the measures described in this book may assist deliberative medical decision making and the avoidance of error, and also find application in other disciplines as well.

# References

1. Aji BM, Larner AJ. Cognitive assessment in an epilepsy clinic using AD8 questionnaire. Epilepsy Behav. 2018;85:234–6.
2. Aji BM, Elhadd K, Larner AJ. Cognitive symptoms in people with epilepsy: role of sleep and mood disturbance. J Sleep Disord Ther. 2019;8:1.
3. Amrhein V, Greenland S, McShane B. Scientists rise up against statistical significance. Nature. 2019;567:305–7.
4. Arroll B, Khin N, Kerse N. Screening for depression in primary care with two verbally asked questions: cross sectional study. BMJ. 2003;327:1144–6.

5. Belmin J, Pariel-Madjlessi S, Surun P, Bentot C, Feteanu D, Lefebvre des Noettes V, et al. The cognitive disorders examination (Codex) is a reliable 3-minute test for detection of dementia in the elderly (validation study in 323 subjects). Presse Med. 2007;36:1183–90.
6. Bharambe V, Larner AJ. Functional cognitive disorders: demographic and clinical features contribute to a positive diagnosis. Neurodegener Dis Manag. 2018;8:377–83.
7. Bland JM, Altman DG. Statistical methods for assessing agreement between two methods of clinical measurement. Lancet. 1986;1:307–10.
8. Borson S, Scanlan J, Brush M, Vitiliano P, Dokmak A. The Mini-Cog: a cognitive "vital signs" measure for dementia screening in multi-lingual elderly. Int J Geriatr Psychiatry. 2000;15:1021–7.
9. Bossuyt PM, Reitsma JB, Bruns DE, et al. The STARD statement for reporting studies of diagnostic accuracy: explanation and elaboration. Clin Chem. 2003;49:7–18.
10. Breiman L, Friedman JH, Olshen RA, Stone CJ. Classification and regression trees. Boca Raton: Taylor & Francis; 1984.
11. Brooke P, Bullock R. Validation of a 6 item cognitive impairment test with a view to primary care usage. Int J Geriatr Psychiatry. 1999;14:936–40.
12. Brown MD, Reeves MJ. Interval likelihood ratios: another advantage for the evidence-based diagnostician. Ann Emerg Med. 2003;42:292–7.
13. Bruffaerts R. Machine learning in neurology: what neurologists can learn from machines and vice versa. J Neurol. 2018;265:2745–8.
14. Burch J, Marson A, Beyer F, et al. Dilemmas in the interpretation of diagnostic accuracy studies on presurgical workup for epilepsy surgery. Epilepsia. 2012;53:1294–302.
15. Cohen J. A coefficient of agreement for nominal scales. Educ Psychol Meas. 1960;20:37–46.
16. Cohen J. Weighted kappa: nominal scale agreement with provision for scaled disagreement or partial credit. Psychol Bull. 1968;70:213–20.
17. Delgado R, Tibau XA. Why Cohen's Kappa should be avoided as performance measure in classification. PLoS One. 2019;14(9):e0222916.
18. De Vet HCW, Mokkink LB, Terwee CB, Hoekstra OS, Knol DL. Clinicians are right not to like Cohen's κ. BMJ. 2013;346:f2515.
19. Edwards A. Note on the "correction for continuity" in testing the significance of the difference between correlated proportions. Psychometrika. 1948;13:185–7.
20. Emblen DJ. Peter Mark Roget. The word and the man. London: Longman; 1970.
21. Fleiss JL. Measuring nominal scale agreement among many raters. Psychol Bull. 1971;76:378–82.
22. Gallagher EJ. The problem with sensitivity and specificity…. Ann Emerg Med. 2003;42:298–303.
23. Galvin JE, Roe CM, Xiong C, Morris JE. Validity and reliability of the AD8 informant interview in dementia. Neurology. 2006;67:1942–8.
24. Galvin JE, Roe CM, Coats MA, Morris JC. Patient's rating of cognitive ability: using the AD8, a brief informant interview, as a self-rating tool to detect dementia. Arch Neurol. 2007;64:725–30.
25. Hsieh S, McGrory S, Leslie F, Dawson K, Ahmed S, Butler CR, et al. The Mini-Addenbrooke's Cognitive Examination: a new assessment tool for dementia. Dement Geriatr Cogn Disord. 2015;39:1–11.
26. Isik AT, Soysal P, Kaya D, Usarel C. Triple test, a diagnostic observation, can detect cognitive impairment in older adults. Psychogeriatrics. 2018;18:98–105.
27. Jenkins CD, Stanton BA, Niemcryk SJ, Rose RM. A scale for the estimation of sleep problems in clinical research. J Clin Epidemiol. 1988;41:313–21.
28. Kahneman D. Thinking, fast and slow. London: Penguin; 2012.
29. Lallukka T, Dregan A, Armstrong D. Comparison of a sleep item from the General Health Questionnaire-12 with the Jenkins Sleep Questionnaire as measures of sleep disturbance. J Epidemiol. 2011;21:474–80.

30. Landis JR, Koch GG. The measurement of observer agreement for categorical data. Biometrics. 1977;33:159–74.
31. Landsheer JA. Impact of prevalence of cognitive impairment on the accuracy of the Montreal Cognitive Assessment. The advantage of using two MoCA thresholds to identify error-prone test scores. Alzheimer Dis Assoc Disord. 2020;34:248–53.
32. Larner AJ. AD8 informant questionnaire for cognitive impairment: pragmatic diagnostic test accuracy study. J Geriatr Psychiatry Neurol. 2015;28:198–202.
33. Larner AJ. MACE versus MoCA: equivalence or superiority? Pragmatic diagnostic test accuracy study. Int Psychogeriatr. 2017;29:931–7.
34. Larner AJ. Dementia screening: a different proposal. Future Neurol. 2018;13:177–9.
35. Larner AJ. MACE for diagnosis of dementia and MCI: examining cut-offs and predictive values. Diagnostics (Basel). 2019;9:E51.
36. Larner AJ. Diagnostic test accuracy studies in dementia. A pragmatic approach. 2nd ed. London: Springer; 2019.
37. Larner AJ. What is test accuracy? Comparing unitary accuracy metrics for cognitive screening instruments. Neurodegener Dis Manag. 2019;9:277–81.
38. Larner AJ. Response to "Triple test, a diagnostic observation, can detect cognitive impairment in older adults". Psychogeriatrics. 2019;19:407–8.
39. Larner AJ. Functional cognitive disorders: update on diagnostic status. Neurodegener Dis Manag. 2020;10:67–72.
40. Larner AJ. Mini-Cog versus Codex (cognitive disorders examination): is there a difference? Dement Neuropsychol. 2020;14:128–33.
41. Larner AJ. Manual of screeners for dementia. Pragmatic test accuracy studies. London: Springer; 2020.
42. Larner AJ. Defining "optimal" test cut-off using global test metrics: evidence from a cognitive screening instrument. Neurodegener Dis Manag. 2020;10:223–30.
43. Larner AJ. Cognitive screening instruments for dementia: comparing metrics of test limitation. medRxiv. 2020; https://doi.org/10.1101/2020.10.29.20222109v1.
44. Larner AJ. Combining results of performance-based and informant test accuracy studies: Bayes or Boole? Dement Geriatr Cogn Disord. 2021;50:29-35.
45. McNemar Q. Note on the sampling error of the difference between correlated proportions or percentages. Psychometrika. 1947;12:153–7.
46. Nasreddine ZS, Phillips NA, Bédirian V, Charbonneau S, Whitehead V, Collin I, et al. The Montreal Cognitive Assessment, MoCA: a brief screening tool for mild cognitive impairment. J Am Geriatr Soc. 2005;53:695–9.
47. National Institute for Health and Care Excellence. Dementia. Assessment, management and support for people living with dementia and their carers. NICE Guideline 97. Methods, evidence and recommendations (https://www.nice.org.uk/guidance/ng97). London: NICE; 2018.
48. Noel-Storr AH, McCleery JM, Richard E, et al. Reporting standards for studies of diagnostic test accuracy in dementia: the STARDdem Initiative. Neurology. 2014;83:364–73.
49. Paradise MB, Glozier NS, Naismith SL, Davenport TA, Hickie IB. Subjective memory complaints, vascular risk factors and psychological distress in the middle-aged: a cross-sectional study. BMC Psychiatry. 2011;11:108.
50. Powers DMW. What the F measure doesn't measure … Features, flaws, fallacies and fixes. arXiv. 2015:1503.06410.2015.
51. Sackett DL, Haynes RB. The architecture of diagnostic research. In: Knottnerus JA, editor. The evidence base of clinical diagnosis. London: BMJ Books; 2002.
52. Schuetz GM, Schlattmann F, Dewey M. Use of 3 × 2 tables with an intention to diagnose approach to assess clinical performance of diagnostic tests: meta-analytical evaluation of coronary CT angiography studies. BMJ. 2012;345:e6717.
53. Song Y, Lu Y. Decision tree methods: applications for classification and prediction. Shanghai Arch Psychiatry. 2015;27:130–5.
54. Stiglitz JE. Measuring what matters. Sci Am. 2020;323(2):20–7.

55. Thiebaut de Schotten M, Foulon C, Nachev P. Brain disconnections link structural connectivity with function and behaviour. Nat Commun. 2020;11:5094.
56. Tversky A, Kahneman D. Advances in prospect theory: cumulative representation of uncertainty. J Risk Uncertain. 1992;5:297–323.
57. Ziso B, Larner AJ. Codex (cognitive disorders examination) decision tree modified for the detection of dementia and MCI. Diagnostics (Basel). 2019;9:E58.

# Index

© Springer Nature Switzerland AG 2021
A. J. Larner, *The 2x2 Matrix*, https://doi.org/10.1007/978-3-030-74920-0